Short
Paediatric
A Revision

;7

To our parents
to whom we owe so much

Commissioning Editor: Ellen Green
Project Development Manager: Jim Killgore
Project Manager: Nancy Arnott
Designer: Erik Bigland

Short Cases for Paediatric Exams
A Revision Guide

Adam W. Glaser
BSc (Hons) MBBS DM MRCP(UK) MRCPCH
Department of Oncology, Great Ormond Street Hospital of Children,
London, UK

John McIntyre
BSc (Hons) MB ChB DM MRCP(UK) MRCPCH
Senior Lecturer in Child Health, Academic Division of Child Health,
Derbyshire Children's Hospital, Derby, UK

Malcolm Battin
MB ChB MRCP(UK) FRCPCH
Senior Lecturer in Neonatology, University of Auckland and
National Women's Hospital, Auckland, NZ

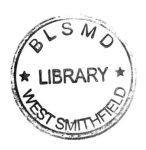

W. B. SAUNDERS

London · Edinburgh · New York · Philadelphia · St Louis · Sydney · Toronto · 2000

W. B. SAUNDERS
An imprint of Harcourt Publishers Limited

© Harcourt Publishers Limited 2000

🅚 is a registered trademark of Harcourt Publishers Limited

First published 2000
  Reprinted 2000

ISBN 0 7020 2162 8

British Library Cataloguing in Publication Data
A catalogue record for this book is available from the British
Library

Library of Congress Cataloging in Publication Data
A catalog record for this book is available from the Library
of Congress

Note
Medical knowledge is constantly changing. As new
information becomes available, changes in treatment,
procedures, equipment and the use of drugs become
necessary. The authors and the publishers have, as far as it is
possible, taken care to ensure that the information given in
this text is accurate and up to date. However, readers are
strongly advised to confirm that the information, especially
with regard to drug usage, complies with the latest
legislation and standards of practice.

The
publisher's
policy is to use
**paper manufactured
from sustainable forests**

Printed in China

Preface

Reaching the clinical section of postgraduate examinations is a major achievement in itself. It will have taken many years of undergraduate training and many dedicated hours of subsequent study, often while doing busy clinical jobs, to get this far. Your knowledge base is broad and considered satisfactory to tackle the final hurdle.

In our experience as both candidates and teachers, it is the short cases that are often the most daunting. Preparing for this section is difficult. The range of possible signs you might see is enormous. The variety of tasks you may be expected to carry out seems never-ending. The potential questions you might have to field seem infinite.

This book may help ease your passage. It is not a comprehensive textbook. We have attempted to cover some 'common' and 'not so common but turn up in exams' cases that appear in short case sections. The emphasis is on the clinical signs that may be seen, with a few key facts to help jog the memory. We have also included brief reminders on how to approach examination of certain systems.

We hope the format of the book will provide a framework for your revision. It is not a substitute for exposure to clinical situations. However, as you see clinical material we hope it will be of use in refining your skills and will stand you in good stead for both the examination you are taking and your future years looking after children.

JMc
MB
AWG

Acknowledgements

The authors gratefully acknowledge the individuals listed below for permission to republish the colour illustrations in the book:

- Figs 1, 3 & 5. Published in *Colour Guide Picture Tests in Neonatology and Paediatrics*. Courtesy of the authors: Warren Hyer, Roslyn Thomas and David Harvey.
- Figs 2, 4 & 7. Published in *Colour Guide Dermatology* 2nd Edition. Courtesy of the authors: J. D. Wilkinson and S. Shaw.
- Fig. 6. Published in *Colour Guide Picture Tests in Ophthalmology*. Courtesy of the authors: J. J. Kanski and K. K. Nischal.

Contents

Contents

Introduction

Short Cases for Paediatric Exams aims to be a revision aid for postgraduate clinical paediatric examinations. Examinations such as The Royal College of Physicians and Child Health (RCPCH) examination in the United Kingdom and Ireland, The Fellowship of the Australian College of Physicians (FRACP) and the Diploma in Child Health (DCH) have a compulsory short case section. Many undergraduates also face an assessment of their clinical skills in a short case setting.

Knowledge of the physical signs found in specific conditions is essential in clinical practice and is also required for examinations. We have endeavoured to put together in a concise format the clinical findings in cases commonly seen in a short case section. The cases are presented in alphabetical order for each system and follow a similar format, where possible, of *physical signs, associations, key points*. We would encourage candidates to use this as a framework and freely add to it their own key points and information that they find helpful. Checklists of what to do when asked to examine a system have been provided in the appendices.

Many candidates find the short case section the most worrying. However, for the well-prepared candidate, the actual experience is rarely as bad as anticipated! For the MRCPCH, a pair of examiners will escort each candidate through the short case section. Often this section is held in a noisy, busy room with many children (and adults) and their accompanying din. It is essential that the candidate remain focused through this. The usual procedure is for one examiner to lead the candidate and ask questions and then the examiners swap over. Do not be put off if they do not appear to encourage you or give you feedback. The examiners follow specific guidelines and will make a detailed report on each candidate.

There is more to the short cases than just eliciting physical signs. In their evaluation, the examiners will assess your approach and attitude to patients; your communication skills with patients; your clinical acumen; your ability to present clinical findings; your ability to solve problems; and your ability to discuss issues. For most candidates we hope this will mean adopting their normal approach: relaxed, friendly but with a confidence that children and parents can respect.

Clinical skills cannot be acquired from reading a book, but rather are learned over time through experience and observing the skilled paediatrician at work. Nevertheless we hope this book will go some way to providing the basic information required for candidates to approach their short cases with confidence.

Respiratory 1

Asthma

Most children with asthma are well between acute exacerbations and the physical examination is normal. Therefore, in short cases, abnormal physical signs are most likely to be of chronic severe asthma or of an acute exacerbation.

Physical signs
- Usually well grown
- Centrally 'pink' at rest
- Determine respiratory rate (usually normal)
- Central trachea
- Comment if chronic chest deformity present, e.g. Harrison's sulci, pectus carinatum, hyperinflation with increased anteroposterior diameter
- Apex beat in normal position
- Symmetrical chest expansion
- Percussion note resonant
- Vesicular breath sounds
- Wheezes and prolonged expiratory phase during acute exacerbation
- Check peak flow in school age child
- Other manifestations of atopy

Associations
- Eczema and allergic rhinitis

Key points
- Childhood asthma is common; prevalence is 10–20% and increasing
- Accounts for 20% of admissions to paediatric wards in school age children
- Hereditary (e.g. atopy) and environmental factors (e.g. viral infections, exposure to allergens, smoking) are important in pathogenesis
- Other respiratory disorders, e.g. cystic fibrosis and bronchopulmonary dysplasia, commonly have an element of reversible obstructive airways disease
- National guidelines published by the British Thoracic Society provide a framework for the management of asthma in childhood

Bronchiectasis

Physical signs
- Productive cough (note if sputum pot is present)
- Often thin and poorly nourished
- Cyanosis may be present in severe cases
- Finger clubbing
- Thoracotomy scar if previous lobectomy
- Chronic chest deformity may be present, e.g. Harrison's sulci
- Coarse crackles, variable wheeze and dull percussion note over the affected area in the presence of secretions.

Associations
- Cystic fibrosis (see p. 7)
- Kartagener's syndrome (see p. 164)
- Hypogammaglobulinaemia

Key points
- Acquired bronchiectasis can occur after childhood pneumonia, measles, whooping cough, tuberculosis and foreign body inhalation
- Management includes treatment of any underlying disorder, physiotherapy and antibiotics during infective episodes
- Surgical removal of the affected area is an option in localised involvement with otherwise relatively good lung function

Bronchopulmonary dysplasia

Physical signs
- Small for corrected age
- May appear cushingoid if on long-term steroid treatment
- Receiving supplemental oxygen, e.g. via nasal cannulae
- Raised respiratory rate
- Intercostal recession
- Vesicular breath sounds with variable wheeze and/or crackles
- Check for signs of pulmonary hypertension and cor pulmonale, e.g. check for single second heart sound, murmur of tricuspid regurgitation, and hepatomegaly

Associations
- Extreme prematurity

Key points
- Need for supplemental O_2 at 28 days with characteristic chest X-ray findings is a useful working definition
- Occurs in 10–20% of surviving preterm infants ventilated for respiratory distress syndrome
- Aetiology unknown, but associations include immaturity, need for O_2 and assisted ventilation, persistent ductus arteriosus, air leaks and infection
- Key aspects of management include providing O_2, ensuring adequate nutrition, treating infections aggressively and supporting the family

Cystic fibrosis

Cystic fibrosis is a multisystem disease and hence the candidate may be required to elicit physical signs in more than one system.

Physical signs
- Comment on nutritional status
- Centrally pink at rest (cyanosis is a late sign)
- Productive cough (look in sputum pot if provided)
- Finger clubbing
- Comment if there is intravenous access (e.g. porta cath, percutaneous long line)

Respiratory
- Respiratory rate (if raised, comment on other signs of respiratory distress, e.g. recession)
- Harrison's sulci, pectus carinatum and hyperinflated chest
- Percussion note resonant (dullness may indicate consolidation or empyema)
- Breath sounds vesicular with variable added sounds – wheezing often present; localised coarse crackles over areas of bronchiectasis
- Nasal polyps
- Peak flow measurement

Abdomen
- Stigmata of chronic liver disease
- Surgical scars (e.g. from meconium ileus, liver transplant)
- Abdominal distension
- Hepatomegaly or splenomegaly, or both
- Faecal masses
- Ascites

Other
- Short stature
- Delayed puberty
- Check injection sites if using insulin

Associations

- Diabetes mellitus in 10% of teenage cases
- Asthma (coexists in about 20% of patients)

Key points

- Autosomal recessive disorder: gene frequency in Caucasians is 1 in 20, and about 1 in 2000 live births is affected
- Cystic fibrosis transmembrane conductance regulator (CFTR) gene is on chromosome 7 (7q31); in the UK, 60% are homozygous for ΔF508 mutation and a further 25% have this on one chromosome and a different mutation on the other
- Neonatal screening available using heel prick sample for immunoreactive trypsin
- Diagnosis confirmed on sweat test
- Management includes regular physiotherapy, antibiotics (prophylaxis and aggressive treatment of infective exacerbations), optimising nutrition, psychosocial support

Interstitial pneumonitis (fibrosing alveolitis)

Physical signs
- Thin
- Non-productive cough
- Finger clubbing
- Possible central cyanosis in advanced cases
- Raised respiratory rate
- Bilateral fine inspiratory crackles at lung bases
- Lung biopsy scar may be present

Associations
- Pulmonary hypertension or cor pulmonale (see p. 21)
- Connective tissue disorders
- Drug reaction

Key points
- Often starts under 5 years of age (50% < 1 year) and cause generally not known
- Chest X-ray shows diffuse hazy ground glass appearance
- Diagnosis made by open lung biopsy
- Children may have an initial symptomatic improvement with steroids

Pleural effusion

Physical signs
- Comment if a drain is in situ
- Raised respiratory rate
- Trachea and apex beat displaced away from the side of the effusion
- Reduced expansion on the affected side
- Percussion note stony dull over effusion
- Reduced or absent breath sounds; bronchial breath sounds are sometimes heard above the effusion level
- Decreased vocal resonance (may be elicited in the older child)

Associations
- Fluid in pleural space may also be chyle (chylothorax), blood (mycobacterium tuberculosis) or pus (empyema)

Key points
- Fluid from a tap should be sent for microscopy, culture (including mycobacterium tuberculosis), protein (transudate <30 g/L; exudate >30 g/L) and cytology
- Causes include:
  — infection, e.g. *Streptococcus pneumoniae*, *Staphylococcus aureus*, tuberculosis
  — hypoalbuminaemia, e.g. nephrotic syndrome
  — malignancy, e.g. lymphoma
  — connective tissue disorders
- Chylothorax can arise from lymphatic drainage problem, e.g. post-cardiac surgery
- Management is supportive, with drainage of fluid and treatment of underlying cause

Pneumonia (lobar)

Physical signs
- In initial stage, patient may look unwell
- Comment on cyanosis and supplemental oxygen if present
- Intravenous cannulae for antibiotics
- Raised respiratory rate
- Use of accessory muscles/intercostal recession
- Central trachea
- Reduced expansion on affected side
- Dull percussion note over area of consolidation
- Bronchial breath sounds over area of consolidation ± coarse crackles
- Vocal resonance increased over affected area

Associations
- Immunodeficiency states

Key points
- Commonest bacterial pathogen is *Streptococcus pneumoniae*
- Clinical improvement is usually rapid with antibiotics
- Pneumococcal empyema may follow and require aspiration

Oesophageal atresia

Oesophageal atresia is commonly associated with other anomalies and may be seen in this context after surgical repair.

Physical signs/associations
- Right lateral thoracotomy scar
- Look at neck for oesphagostomy site and abdomen for gastrostomy

Associated anomalies
V – vertebral: hemi- or bifid vertebrae
  hypersegmentation (13–14 ribs ± thoracic vertebrae; 6–7 lumbar vertebrae)
A – anal: anorectal malformation
C – cardiac: ventricular septal defect, tetralogy of Fallot (see p. 24 and p. 23)
T – trachea: tracheo-oesophageal fistula
E – oesophageal: oesophageal atresia
R – renal: hydronephrosis, renal dysplasia, vesicoureteric reflux
L – limb: radial dysplasia

Key points
- Incidence of ~1:3000–4000 and equal sex ratio
- Antenatal diagnosis may be suggested by polyhydramnios with skeletal, cardiac and renal anomalies; postnatal presentation may be with bubbly saliva, choking or aspiration on attempted feeding
- 85% with oesophageal atresia have a distal tracheo-oesophageal fistula and ~ 7% have atresia without a fistula
- Standard treatment is primary repair of oesophagus with closure of the fistula
- Long-term problems include anastomotic stricture, dysmotility, gastro-oesophageal reflux, respiratory symptoms

Stridor

Physical signs
- Comment on age and general condition of the child
- Stridor is usually inspiratory; can be expiratory (narrowing severe or in lower trachea)
- Determine quality of the voice: hoarseness or weakness implies glottic involvement
- Examine neck and chest for signs of increased work of breathing, surgical scars and clues to aetiology

Causes

Chronic	Acute
Laryngomalacia	Croup
Micrognathia	(laryngotracheobronchitis)
Laryngeal web, polyp or papilloma	Epiglottitis
Laryngeal cleft	Foreign body
Vocal cord paralysis	Angioneurotic oedema
Subglottic stenosis	Hypocalcaemic tetany
Haemangioma	Diphtheria
Vascular ring	
Foreign body	

Key points
- Age, duration of symptoms and clinical findings often point to the diagnosis
- Laryngomalacia is the commonest cause in infancy; stridor is usually present shortly after birth
- Investigations for chronic stridor include chest and neck X-ray (foreign body), barium swallow (vascular ring) and laryngoscopy/bronchoscopy
- Indications for further investigation include persistent severe stridor, failure to thrive, recurrent choking

Cardiovascular

2

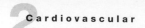

Aortic stenosis

Physical signs
- Well grown
- Centrally pink
- Brachial pulses are often small volume and slow rising; plateau in type but may be normal
- Forceful pulsation of the left ventricle
- Systolic thrill in suprasternal notch
- Ejection systolic murmur loudest over second right intercostal space and at cardiac apex; radiates to the neck over the carotid arteries
- Often an ejection click precedes the murmur and is best heard at the apex during expiration
- Aortic second heart sound is soft and delayed
- Paradoxical splitting of second heart sound may occur in severe stenosis

Associations
- William syndrome
- Turner syndrome

Key points
- Accounts for about 5% of congenital heart lesions and is more common in boys
- Aortic valve is commonly bicuspid with partial fusion of commissures, but it may be unicusped or non-cusped
- Obstruction may occur above the valve (supravalvular stenosis – see William syndrome, p. 176) or below (subvalvular – due to fibrous diaphragm)
- Aortic stenosis is usually asymptomatic, but when severe it may present in infancy with heart failure or sudden death, or in older children with effort syncope
- Valvotomy is required for severe stenosis, but if possible valve replacement should be postponed until adult life

Atrial septal defect (primum)

Physical signs
- Centrally pink
- Often breathless at rest: look for signs of increased work of breathing, e.g. intercostal recession or chronic chest deformity (e.g. Harrison's sulci)
- Normal brachial pulses
- Displaced apex beat
- Right ventricular heave
- Fixed splitting of the second heart sound
- Soft ejection systolic murmur loudest at the second left intercostal space
- Harsh pansystolic murmur loudest at the apex radiating to the axilla

Associations
- Down syndrome (see p. 156)

Key points
- Often present with failure to thrive and heart failure in infancy
- Defect occurs in the lowest part of the atrial septum, with a cleft in the anterior leaflet of the mitral valve
- Apical murmur is due to mitral regurgitation
- ECG findings are left axis deviation, biventricular hypertrophy and incomplete bundle branch block
- Treatment is early surgery to close the defect and repair the valve

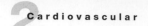

Atrial septal defect (secundum)

Physical signs
- Pink and well grown
- Normal brachial pulses
- Right ventricular heave
- Fixed splitting of the second heart sound
- Soft ejection systolic murmur loudest at the second left intercostal space

Associations
- Noonan syndrome (see p. 168)
- Holt–Oram syndrome (see p. 162)

Key points
- Accounts for about 8% of congenital defects
- With a large shunt there may also be a diastolic murmur in the tricuspid area
- Rarely causes symptoms in childhood, but untreated it may present with pulmonary hypertension, heart failure or arrhythmias in early adult life
- Treatment is surgical, using cardiopulmonary bypass with either direct suturing or a patch
- ECG demonstrates normal or right axis deviation, right bundle branch block and usually right ventricular hypertrophy (compare with primum atrial septal defect)

Coarctation of the aorta (older children)

Physical signs
- Centrally pink and well grown
- Normal brachial pulses
- Weak or absent femoral pulses
- Femoral pulses may be palpable but delayed in the older child where collateral circulation has been established
- Elevated blood pressure in the right arm with reduced systolic and pulse pressure in the legs
- Normal heart sounds
- An ejection systolic murmur is often heard best at the back between the scapulae
- Collateral vessels may be palpable in the intercostal spaces on the medial borders of the scapulae

Associations
- Turner syndrome (see p. 172)
- Other cardiovascular abnormalities, e.g. ventricular septal defect, bicuspid aortic valve, mitral valve abnormalities

Key points
- Infants with severe coarctation present with heart failure as the ductus arteriosus closes
- The constriction usually occurs just distal to the origin of the left subclavian artey
- Occasionally the narrowing is above the origin of the left subclavian artery, giving rise to weak pulses and reduced systolic blood pressure in the left arm
- Treatment is by surgical repair, often using a subclavian flap operation, resulting in absent or reduced left upper limb pulses
- Balloon dilatation can be used if re-stenosis occurs

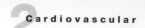

Patent ductus arteriosus

Physical signs
- Centrally pink
- Brachial pulses collapsing in character
- Wide pulse pressure
- Apex beat displaced
- Thrill felt in first and second left intercostal spaces
- Continuous 'machinery' murmur loudest at second left intercostal space radiating to below the left clavicle; reaches maximal intensity towards the end of systole and fades away in diastole
- A mid-diastolic murmur may be heard at the apex due to increased flow across a normal mitral valve

Associations
- Down's syndrome
- Congenital rubella

Key points
- A persistent ductus arteriosus is common in extremely premature babies; unlike in mature infants, it is often managed successfully with fluid restriction and indomethacin
- In mature infants, it accounts for about 7% of congenital heart lesions
- A small ductus arteriosus is likely to be asymptomatic; with increasing size of shunt there may be poor weight gain, reduced exercise tolerance or heart failure
- Conventional treatment is by surgical ligation; occlusion with an 'umbrella' inserted via a catheter is increasingly being used

Pulmonary hypertension

Physical signs
- Mild central cyanosis
- Finger clubbing
- Normal brachial pulse
- Right ventricular heave
- Loud second heart sound in the pulmonary area that may be palpable
- Short ejection systolic murmur in pulmonary area often preceded by an ejection click

Key points
- With established pulmonary hypertension, there is gradually increasing cyanosis and heart failure
- The 'Eisenmenger complex' describes large ventricular septal defects with right-to-left shunts producing cyanosis
- Eisenmenger's syndrome describes pulmonary hypertension at systemic level due to pulmonary vascular resistance with reversed or bidirectional shunting
- Pulmonary hypertension may be primary (idiopathic); it may be secondary to congenital heart defects with increased pulmonary blood flow or raised pulmonary venous pressure
- Heart–lung transplantation is a possible treatment option

Pulmonary stenosis

Physical signs
- Centrally pink
- Well grown
- Normal brachial pulses
- Apex beat 'tapping' in quality
- Parasternal heave of right ventricular hypertrophy
- Systolic thrill in the second left intercostal space
- Ejection click may be heard
- Harsh ejection systolic murmur loudest over the second left intercostal space, radiating to the lung apex
- Splitting of the second heart sound widens with increasing severity of stenosis

Associations
- Noonan syndrome (see p. 168)
- William syndrome (see p. 176)

Key points
- Isolated pulmonary stenosis accounts for ~ 8% of congenital heart disease
- In mild stenosis, the right ventricular–pulmonary artery pressure gradient is <30 mmHg and no treatment is required apart from antibiotic prophylaxis
- The pressure gradient is >60 mmHg in severe stenosis
- Balloon dilatation valvuloplasty is now the preferred treatment
- Severe stenosis can present in infancy with cyanosis (due to right-to-left shunt at the atrial level through the foramen ovale) and heart failure

Tetralogy of Fallot

Physical signs
- Centrally pink in early infancy; cyanosis usually present by the end of the first year
- Finger clubbing may be present
- Normal brachial pulses
- Normal apex beat
- Systolic thrill in pulmonary area
- Ejection systolic murmur loudest at the second left intercostal space
- Single second heart sound

Association
- Down syndrome (see p. 156)

Key points
- Accounts for about 5% of congenital defects
- The four abnormalities are: stenosis of the pulmonary valve or infundibulum; ventricular septal defect; hypertrophy of the right ventricle; overriding aorta
- Complications to be aware of are cerebral thrombosis, cerebral abscess, bacterial endocarditis and haemorrhagic tendency
- 'Cyanotic spells' due to decreased pulmonary blood flow can occur following crying or exertion; 'squatting' may increase systemic vascular resistance, reduce venous return from the legs and improve pulmonary blood flow
- Timing and type of surgical treatment depend on the clinical severity of the lesion
- Palliative shunt procedure (e.g. Blalock–Taussig operation) may be required if the right ventricular outflow tract is poorly developed before later definitive surgery

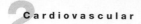

Ventricular septal defect

Physical signs

Small defect
- Centrally pink
- Well grown
- Normal pulses
- Apex beat is undisplaced
- Systolic thrill may be present and is maximal at 3rd and 4th intercostal spaces at the left sternal edge
- Normal heart sounds
- Harsh pansystolic murmur maximal at the lower left sternal edge
- No signs of cardiac failure

Large defect
- Centrally pink
- Poorly nourished
- Breathless at rest with signs of increased work of breathing
- Normal pulses
- Displaced apex beat, thrusting quality
- Parasternal heave
- Systolic thrill maximal at 3rd and 4th intercostal spaces at the left sternal edge
- Heart sounds may be normal; second sound may become loud and single in large defect with pulmonary hypertension
- Harsh pansystolic murmur maximal at the lower left sternal edge radiating widely
- Mid-diastolic murmur at apex (from increased flow across mitral valve)
- Hepatomegaly

Associations
- Chromosomal abnormalities, e.g. trisomy 18, 21, cri du chat syndrome
- Syndromes, e.g. Holt–Oram, de Lange syndrome, VACTERL

Key points

- Most common congenital heart lesion accounting for approximately one-third of cases
- Usually 'multifactorial inheritance'; recurrence risk if one child affected ~ 3%
- Outcome depends on the size of the defect and position in the septum; small defects in the muscular part of the septum are more likely to close than large defects in the perimembranous area
- Small defects without significant haemodynamic changes require no treatment other than antibiotic prophylaxis
- With large defects, primary surgical closure before pulmonary hypertension is established is usually possible

Abdomen

Chronic liver disease

Physical signs
- Jaundice
- Cyanosis, if pulmonary venous shunting is present
- Failure to thrive and cachexia
- Clubbing and leuconychia
- Palmar erythema
- Dupuytren's contracture
- Small muscle wasting
- Bruising due to vitamin K deficiency
- Excoriations – deposited bile pigments cause itching
- Xanthomata over extensor surfaces and sites of pressure
- Signs of vitamin D deficiency – rickety rosary and epiphyseal widening
- Gynaecomastia
- Spider naevi
- Abdominal scars suggesting previous Kasai procedure
- Distended abdominal veins
- Hepatomegaly – may not be present if cirrhosis is established
- Splenomegaly, if portal hypertension is present
- Ascites
- Oedema – this is dependent in older children but commonly periorbital or around the arms in younger children
- Encephalopathy with altered conscious state
- Other signs associated with underlying cause, e.g. cystic fibrosis or Wilson's disease

Causes
- Cystic fibrosis (see p. 7)
- Biliary atresia
- Choledochal cyst
- Total parenteral nutrition
- Wilson disease (see p. 40)
- Galactosaemia
- Hereditary fructose intolerance

- Alpha-1-antitrypsin deficiency
- Tyrosinaemia
- Viral hepatitis
- Autoimmune chronic active hepatitis
- Alagille syndrome (see p. 146)
- Drugs, including isoniazid and methotrexate

Chronic renal disease

Physical signs
- Failure to thrive
- Pallor/sallow complexion
- Bruising and petechiae
- Brown lines on nails
- Small muscle wasting
- Wrist flaring, rickety rosary and bow legs due to abnormal vitamin D metabolism
- Arteriovenous fistula if requiring haemodialysis
- Hypertension
- Congestive cardiac failure – elevated jugular venous pressure, third heart sound, hepatomegaly, oedema
- Abdominal scars from continuous ambulatory peritoneal dialysis (CAPD)
- Abdominal mass, including renal masses or renal transplants in iliac fossae
- Delayed pubertal development
- Urinalysis – albumin, blood, pH and specific gravity
- Other signs of underlying pathology

Causes
- Congenital anomalies, including hypoplasia, obstruction and other malformations
- Inherited conditions such as polycystic kidneys and Alport syndrome (nephritis and sensorineural deafness)
- Acquired glomerular disorders, including haemolytic uraemic syndrome and glomerulonephritis

Coeliac disease (gluten-sensitive enteropathy)

Physical signs
- Short stature
- Decreased subcutaneous fat and muscle wasting, particularly of the proximal limbs and buttocks
- Pallor
- Glossitis
- Finger clubbing may be present
- Dermatitis herpetiformis: erythematous papules with excoriations ± vesicles
- Peripheral oedema
- Abdominal distension

Associations
- Diabetes mellitus – incidence of coeliac disease increased 50-fold (see p. 132)
- Chronic liver disease (see p. 28)
- Autoimmune disorders may occur
- Lymphoma of the small intestine in middle age
- IgA deficiency

Key points
- Incidence is 1:2–3000; in certain areas it is higher, e.g. west coast of Ireland
- Associated with HLA-A1, -B8 and -DR3 haplotypes
- Siblings and offspring have a 10% risk of developing coeliac disease
- Serological tests (antigliadin, antireticulin and endomysial antibodies) are increasingly used. Diagnosis is made on characteristic small bowel biopsy histology, which then returns to normal on a gluten-free diet
- Gluten-free diet is recommended for life

Hepatomegaly, splenomegaly and hepatosplenomegaly

HEPATOMEGALY

Physical signs
- Mass in the right subcostal area, which may extend across the midline
- Cannot feel between the mass and the costal margin
- Moves down towards the right iliac fossa on inspiration
- Describe if uniform or irregular enlargement and whether smooth or firm
- Define the degree of enlargement by measuring the distance it extends below the right costal margin in the midclavicular line
- Examine for associated splenomegaly and ascites
- Search for signs of chronic liver disease (see p. 28) and causes of hepatomegaly
- Check that patient is not in congestive cardiac failure

Causes

Infection
- Viral
  - hepatitis A/B/C/D/E
  - cytomegalovirus
  - Epstein–Barr
- Bacterial
  - septicaemia
  - tuberculosis
- Parasitic
  - malaria
  - toxoplasmosis
  - hydatid

Metabolic/storage miscellaneous
- Defect in carbohydrate metabolism
  - glycogen storage diseases (see p. 135)
  - galactosaemia
- Defect in lipid metabolism
  - Gaucher disease
- Defect in protein metabolism
  - tyrosinaemia
  - extrahepatic biliary atresia
  - alpha-1-antitrypsin deficiency
  - Wilson disease (see p. 40)
- Inflammatory
  - associated with inflammatory bowel disease, connective tissue disorders

Haematological
- Haemolytic disease of the newborn
- Thalassaemia (see p. 129)
- Sickle cell disease (see p. 127)

Malignancy
- Lymphoma
- Leukaemia
- Primary liver tumour, e.g. hepatoblastoma
- Secondary deposits, e.g. from neuroblastoma

Cardiac
- Heart failure

SPLENOMEGALY

Physical signs
- Mass in left subcostal region
- Cannot feel between the mass and the costal margin
- Moves down and across the abdomen towards the right iliac fossa on inspiration
- Notched surface can be felt
- Mass is not ballottable on bimanual palpation (c.f. kidney)

- Define the degree of enlargement by measuring the maximum distance it extends below the left costal margin
- Examine for associated hepatomegaly and ascites
- Examine for signs suggestive of portal hypertension, including chronic liver disease, dilated veins on surface of abdomen
- Search for signs of chronic liver disease (see p. 28) and causes of splenomegaly

Causes

Infection
- Viral
  - Epstein–Barr virus
  - cytomegalovirus
- Bacterial
  - septicaemia
  - subacute bacterial endocarditis
- Parasitic
  - malaria
  - toxoplasmosis

Metabolic/miscellaneous
- Gaucher disease (see p. 134)
- Connective tissue disease
  - juvenile chronic arthritis (see p. 110)
  - systemic lupus erythematosus(see p. 115)

Haematological
- Chronic haemolytic anaemia
  - hereditary spherocytosis

Malignancy
- Lymphoma
- Leukaemia

Portal hypertension
- Hepatocellular disease
  - Wilson's disease (see p. 40)
  - alpha-1-antitrypsin deficiency

- Biliary tract disease, e.g. extrahepatic biliary atresia
- Portal vein occlusion
- Budd–Chiari syndrome

HEPATOSPLENOMEGALY

Physical signs
- Signs of enlarged liver and spleen (see above)
- Signs of portal hypertension
- Examine for ascites
- Stigmata of chronic liver disease

Causes
The causes of hepatomegaly and splenomegaly outline the range of possibilities:

- infection – Epstein–Barr virus, cytomegalovirus, rubella, hepatitis, toxoplasmosis
- metabolic – mucopolysaccharidoses, alpha-1-antitrypsin deficiency (see p. 139)
- haematological – thalassaemia (see p. 129)
- malignancy – lymphoma, leukaemia.

Nephrotic syndrome

Physical signs
- Oedema – around the ankle and legs in older children; in younger children may present with periorbital oedema
- Abdominal distension – ascites and/or hepatomegaly may be present
- Pleural effusion
- Check blood pressure – normal in most children but there may be postural hypotension or mild hypertension (15%)
- Proteinuria (ask to check urine if this diagnosis is suspected)
- Other features that may occur:
  — white bands across nails (due to chronic hypoalbuminaemia)
  — tendon xanthomata or orbital xanthelasmata (due to hypercholesterolaemia)
  — cushingoid features secondary to therapeutic corticosteroids

Associations
- Pneumococcal peritonitis or cellulitis
- Hypercoagulability leading to thromboses and emboli
- Hypercholesterolaemia

Key points
- Male to female ratio of 2:1
- 90% due to minimal change nephrotic syndrome; other causes are focal segmental glomerulosclerosis, mesangiocapillary glomerulonephritis, membranous glomerulonephritis or systemic lupus erythematosus
- 50–80% of minimal change cases show a relapsing course
- Corticosteroids are first-line therapy – 85% lose proteinuria within 4 weeks
- Steroid-sparing drugs used include cyclophosphamide, levamisole and cyclosporin

Prune belly syndrome

Physical signs
- Usually male
- Deficient abdominal wall musculature with skin hanging in wrinkled folds
- Distended abdomen
- Kidneys may be palpable due to hydronephrosis
- Check blood pressure (as renal involvement)
- Cryptorchidism

Associations
- Cardiac abnormalities, e.g. ventricular septal defect, atrial septal defect
- Musculoskeletal defects, e.g. talipes, congenital dislocation of the hips
- Pulmonary hypoplasia

Key points
- ~ 3% are female
- Usually sporadic with less than 1% recurrence risk for siblings
- Treatment aims to prevent urinary tract infections and optimise renal tract drainage

Renal enlargement

Physical signs
- Deep flank mass – ballottable on bimanual palpation, can get above it on palpation; percussion note resonant
- Arteriovenous fistula (if patient is requiring haemodialysis)
- Elevated blood pressure
- Hypertensive retinopathy
- Urinalysis – blood, albumin, pH and specific gravity
- Associated genitourinary abnormalities (e.g. WAGA – Wilms' and genitourinary abnormalities)
- Hepatomegaly in infantile polycystic disease
- Other signs of underlying pathology, e.g. tuberous sclerosis or glycogen storage disease

Causes

Unilateral renal enlargement
- Hydronephrosis
- Renal cyst
- Tumours – Wilms' tumour, renal cell carcinoma, congenital mesoblastic nephroma, neuroblastoma, phaeochromocytoma

Bilateral renal enlargement
- Polycystic renal disease – the infant form is autosomal recessively inherited and associated with cystic disease of other organs, especially the liver; the adult form is autosomal dominantly inherited
- Hydronephrosis – in boys, consider posterior urethral valves. Other causes include neurogenic bladder, e.g. children with spina bifida, or vesicoureteric reflux
- Wilms' tumour, bilateral in 10%
- Tuberous sclerosis (see p. 91)
- Glycogen storage disease types 1a and 1b (see p. 135)
- Amyloidosis (rare in children)

Renal transplant

Physical signs
- Mass in right iliac fossa
- Scars from central venous lines and arteriovenous fistulae previously used for dialysis
- Hypertrichosis due to cyclosporin used to prevent rejection
- Hypertension secondary to steroids, cyclosporin or previous renal disease
- Cushingoid features due to long-term steroid use
- Failure to thrive and delayed sexual development secondary to preceding end-stage renal failure and drugs to prevent rejection

Associations
- Features of underlying pathology resulting in end-stage renal failure, e.g. systemic lupus erythematosus (see p. 115), Alport's syndrome, cystinosis

Key features
- Significant morbidity associated with immunosuppressive drugs
- Post-transplant complications include recurrence of underlying pathology, infections, rejection, drug toxicity, acute tubular necrosis
- Psychosocial and supportive care, including growth hormone replacement therapy, enhance rehabilitation

Wilson disease (hepatolenticular degeneration)

Physical signs
- Jaundice
- Anaemia
- Kayser–Fleischer rings – rim of brown pigment at edge of iris
- Hepatomegaly or hepatosplenomegaly
- Neurological abnormalities, e.g. slurred speech; other features, such as choreoathetosis, resting and intention tremor, dystonia and myoclonus, are rare in childhood
- Stigmata of chronic liver disease (p. 28)
- Change in personality and psychotic behaviour

Associations
- Chronic active hepatitis
- Vitamin-D-resistant rickets

Key points
- Autosomal recessive inheritance; gene on chromosome 13
- Incidence is 30 per 1 million population
- Disorder of copper metabolism with reduced biliary copper excretion, lowered plasma caeruloplasmin and raised urinary copper excretion
- Treatment of choice is D-penicillamine, with trientine as an alternative

Nervous system

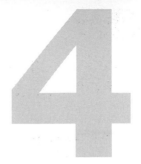

Ataxia telangiectasia

Physical signs
- Telangiectasia on bulbar conjunctiva, bridge of nose and auricles
- Progressive ataxia: initially truncal but subsequently involves gait
- Intention tremor
- Choreoathetosis
- Nystagmus
- Altered skin pigmentation and café-au-lait patches
- Signs of frequent respiratory infection, e.g. bronchiectasis (p. 5)
- Failure to thrive

Associations
- Defective DNA repair leads to high incidence of lymphoreticular malignancy
- Immune deficiency with hypogammaglobulinaemia in more than 50%

Key points
- Autosomal recessive; gene defect on chromosome 11
- Diagnosis confirmed by chromosome fragility
- No curative treatment
- Management involves treatment of infection and chemotherapy for malignancies
- Ionising radiation should be avoided
- Child often wheelchair-bound in adolescence
- Life span is dependent on infections and neoplasia

Cerebral palsy

Physical signs

- Posture may be hemiplegic, diplegic or 'windswept' in severe quadriplegia
- Test tone, power and reflexes in all four limbs
- Comment on:
  - — any abnormal movements
  - — the presence of joint contractures or weakness
  - — the presence of orthosis, splints or wheelchair
  - — vasomotor changes: affected limbs may be cool with peripheral cyanosis
- Brisk tendon jerks and extensor plantars are usually present
- Head circumference should be measured, as either hydrocephalus or microcephaly may be present
- Note weight and height/length so as to comment on growth and nutritional status
- Scoliosis
- Gait analysis if appropriate; subtle degrees of altered tone may need to be elicted by stressing gait
- Abnormal eye movements
- Strabismus
- Visual field defects
- Blindness or optic atrophy

Associations

- Mental retardation in up to 50%
- Squint in 30%
- Seizures in 30%
- Visual impairment

Key points

- Cerebral palsy is defined as a permanent non-progressive disorder of posture and movement due to an insult to developing brain. Although the lesion is non-progressive, the clinical picture may evolve over time
- Patterns of cerebral palsy include spastic (70%), ataxic, athetoid and mixed
- Prevalence approximately 2 in 1000 live births
- The aetiology includes:
  — prenatal, e.g. placental dysfunction, drug exposure or infection
  — perinatal, e.g. hypoxia, haemorrhage
  — postnatal, e.g. trauma or infection
- Management requires a multidisiplinary approach

Charcot–Marie–Tooth (hereditary motor sensory neuropathy I, peroneal muscular atrophy)

Physical signs
- Characteristic 'inverted champagne bottle' contour to lower limbs due to atrophy of the anterior compartment muscles
- Bilateral progressive weakness of ankle dorsiflexion and eventual foot drop
- Pes cavus
- Abnormal gait with slapping of feet, frequent tripping and falls
- Loss of distal deep tendon reflexes (ankle ± knee)
- Upper limb reflexes preserved
- Upper limbs may be affected, but atrophy of muscles in the forearm is usually a late finding
- Contractures of the wrists and fingers may produce a claw hand
- Sensory involvement – initially loss of proprioception and vibration sense; pain and temperature sensation affected late in disease and may result in callus or pressure areas on feet
- Affected nerves become palpably enlarged (check ulnar, radial and peroneal)
- Autonomic effects, e.g. cold feet with blotching or pallor of the skin
- Sphincter control, cardiac, gastrointestinal and bladder control are preserved
- Kyphoscoliosis
- Normal cranial nerves

Association
- Sensory neural hearing loss

Key points
- Age of onset is bimodal but early peak occurs in first two decades and signs may appear before 1 year
- Inheritance is autosomal dominant, with males and females equally affected
- Prevalence is 3.8 in 100 000

- Disease onset is usually in adolescence but is variable from childhood upwards
- Nerve conduction velocity is decreased in motor and sensory nerves and is usually seen in one parent
- Management includes genetic counselling, physiotherapy, foot stabilisation and special adaptive devices for hands if affected
- Prognosis is a normal life span and most patients remain ambulant
- Hereditary motor sensory neuropathy (HMSN) type II has a similar clinical picture but slower progression
- HMSN type III patients have massive 'onion bulb' nerve hypertrophy and may demonstrate facial weakness, kyphoscoliosis, pes cavus and marked muscle atrophy. Onset is early in life and milestones may be delayed but intelligence is normal

Cranial nerve palsy

THIRD CRANIAL NERVE PALSY

Physical signs
- Ptosis (complete or partial)
- Retract lid – eye is deviated down and out
- Impaired adduction and elevation of eye
- Pupil may be dilated

SIXTH NERVE CRANIAL PALSY

Physical signs
- Failure of lateral abduction of eye
- Maximal diplopia on looking to affected side
- Images parallel and separated horizontally
- Head may turn to side of affected muscle to limit diplopia

Associations
Causes of ophthalmoplegia include:

- brainstem encephalitis
- mononeuritis multiplex
- midbrain vascular lesions or haemorrhage
- migraine
- meningitis
- Miller–Fisher syndrome (ataxia, external opthalmoplegia and areflexia)
- myasthenia gravis
- direct involvement with tumour or aneurysm

Key point
- Sixth nerve palsy is a false localising sign in raised intracranial pressure

FACIAL PALSY

Physical signs
- Mouth sags
- Asymmetrical smile

- Drooling of mouth
- Difficulty in blowing out cheeks
- Incomplete closure of eye
- Wrinkling forehead is relatively preserved in upper motor neurone lesion, but in lower motor neurone involvement the upper and lower face are equally affected
- Associated features vary with site of lesion and include loss of taste on anterior two-thirds of tongue or hyperacusis

Causes
- Birth injury
- Idiopathic or postviral
- Infective, e.g. Epstein–Barr, herpes simplex, mumps
- Trauma, e.g. fracture of temporal bone
- Space-occupying lesion

Key points
- Symptoms due to minor birth trauma usually resolve
- Bell palsy: acute isolated unilateral facial palsy of undetermined cause
  - 80% make complete recovery in 3 months
  - 10% have residual mild facial weakness
  - 5% have permanent severe facial weakness
  - Treatment is to protect eye ± short course of prednisolone 2 mg/kg per day

Duchenne muscular dystrophy

Physical signs
Signs vary considerably with age.

- In a young boy, initial signs include difficulty climbing stairs and lumbar lordosis; signs are subtle and may be overlooked
- In an older boy, signs are more marked with pseudohypertrophy of calves or deltoid
- Wasting of pelvic girdle and back
- Contractures of the Achilles tendon occur early
- Weakness is most marked proximally
- Facial muscles are spared weakness
- Tendon reflexes may become depressed
- Gower's manoeuvre when getting off floor (ask examiner prior to demonstration so as not to fatigue child)
- Initially toe walking gait with frequent falls
- Subsequently waddling gait (Trendelenburg sign is positive, i.e. the hip drops down when the ipsilateral foot is raised)
- An older boy may use walking calipers or a wheelchair

Associations
- Cardiomyopathy in 50–80%
- Scoliosis
- Mental retardation: mean IQ is 85

Key points
- X-linked recessive inheritance
- One-third have new mutations
- Incidence is 1 in 4000 male births
- Onset is usually within 3 years of birth
- Diagnosis is made on elevated CPK, myopathic EMG and characteristic findings on muscle biopsy
- Female carrier is non-symptomatic but may have pseudohypertrophy and weakness of pelvic girdle
- Despite supportive treatment, including night ventilation, prognosis is poor with death in the second decade

Floppy baby

Physical signs

- Note posture – a hypotonic infant will adopt a 'frog's leg' position when supine
- Spontaneous movements may be present and should be commented on
- Comment on face, including dysmorphic features (Down or Prader–Will), facial movements and alertness (SMA characteristically alert)
- Joint contractures indicate long-standing inactivity
- Muscles may appear soft and flabby with excessive range of passive movement in congenital myopathies
- Head lag – demonstrated by pulling to sit (but support head when doing this)
- Head control poor when held upright
- Truncal tone is decreased; demonstrated by holding in ventral suspension/prone
- Decreased tone demonstrated in hip adduction, popliteal angle, ankle flexion and 'scarf sign'
- Tendon reflexes may be diminished or exaggerated depending on the disease process

Classification of causes of hypotonia

- Cerebral – benign congenital hypotonia, cerebral malformation, hypoxic ischaemic encephalopathy
- Chromosomal disorders – Down syndrome, Prader–Willi syndrome
- Metabolic defects – Zellweger syndrome
- Genetic – familial dysautonomia, Lowe syndrome
- Neonatal spinal cord injury – difficult delivery
- Motor neurone disorders – spinal muscular atrophy, infantile neuronal degeneration, incontinentia pigmenti
- Disorders of neuromuscular transmission – infantile botulism, myasthenia gravis
- Myopathies – centronuclear, nemaline rod, central core
- Muscular dystrophies – congenital muscular dystrophy, myotonic dystrophy

- Metabolic myopathies – acid maltase deficiency, carnitine deficiency, phosphofructokinase deficiency, phosphorylase deficiency
- Infantile myositis

Key points

Investigation depends on clinical findings but may include karyotype, chromosome studies, metabolic screen, cerebral imaging, EMG and muscle biopsy.

Friedreich ataxia

Physical signs
- Progressive ataxia with gait disturbance
- Cerebellar dysfunction
  - dysarthria
  - dysdiadochokinesia
  - finger–nose ataxia
  - head titubation
  - positive Romberg's test
- Tone normal or reduced
- Distal weakness affecting lower limbs more than upper
- Extensor plantar responses
- Absent knee and ankle reflexes
- Distal loss of joint position and vibration, particularly in lower limbs
- Hammer toes;
- Pes cavus
- Progressive kyphoscoliosis
- Optic atrophy
- Lateral gaze nystagmus
- Neurosensory hearing loss

Associations
- Arrhythmias
- Hypertrophic cardiomyopathy (60–90%)
- Diabetes mellitus (10–25%)

Key points
- Incidence – 1 in 100 000 live births
- Most common spinocerebellar degeneration
- Age of onset usually 8–15 years
- Inheritance is usually autosomal recessive with defect localised to chromosome 9
- Early ECG changes are inverted T-waves or signs of left ventricular hypertrophy

Guillain–Barré syndrome

Physical signs
- Hypotonia
- Weakness is usually symmetrical and more marked distally
- Trunk and bulbar musculature may be affected in established cases
- Areflexia or hyporeflexia – usually symmetrical but may initially be asymmetrical
- Sensory deficits include loss of position/vibratory sensation before pain and touch
- Cranial nerve palsies are present in ~30% and may occur at any time
- All cranial nerves may be affected although olfactory involvement is rare; facial nerve involvement is most common, ~50%; dysphagia (9th and 10th) is second most common
- If there is extraocular muscle involvement, think of Miller–Fisher syndrome (ataxia, external ophthalmoplegia and areflexia)
- Comment on sweating or flushing and ask to measure BP, check peak flow and examine cardiovascular system

Associations
- Autonomic dysfunction – sweating, hypertension, orthostatic hypotension and tachyarrhythmias
- Respiratory failure – respiratory paralysis occurs in up to 20% of untreated cases

Key points
- GB occurs at any age in childhood, but peak is 4–7 years
- Insidious symptoms of sensory deficit, pain or paraesthesia may precede motor weakness
- Nerve conduction velocity reduced and EMG consistent with lower motor neurone deficit
- Treatment with plasmapheresis or immunoglobulins may be beneficial
- Ventilation is indicated for respiratory failure, cardiovascular instability and, if progression to dysphagia, shoulder or facial paresis
- Prognosis – 3–4% mortality; 50% recover within 6 months; 10% with permanent deficits; 7% relapse

Horner's syndrome

Physical signs
- Ptosis
- Miosis – best seen in dim light so normal pupil dilates
- Anhidrosis of ipsilateral side of face
- Enophthalmos
- Congenital cases may show heterochromia of iris

Associations
Sympathetic denervation of the eye caused by:

- brachial plexus damage at birth
- neuroblastoma or other childhood tumours in mediastinum or cervical region
- injury to superior cervical ganglion or sympathetic trunk, e.g. post-surgical
- congenital factors – autosomal dominant.

Macrocephaly

Physical signs
- Large head – measure and plot occipital–frontal circumference (OFC); > 3 standard deviations
- In neonate or infant, full fontanelle, widened sutures and sun setting of eyes suggest hydrocephalus
- In older children, 'cracked pot sound' on percussion of skull suggests separation of sutures
- In *all children* look for:
  — ventriculoperitoneal shunt/surgical scars
  — signs of raised intracranial pressure (acute cases not likely in exam)
  — cranial bruit – vein of Galen malformations
  — dysmorphism, e.g. mucopolysaccharidosis (see p. 139)
  — thickened skull in thalassaemia or osteopetrosis
  — skeletal abnormalities or evidence of spina bifida
  — ask to check vision/eye movements/fundi
  — measure parents' OFC and plot height/weight centiles

Causes
- Familial macrocephaly (see p. 55)
- Achondroplasia (see p. 108)
- Sotos syndrome (see p. 139)
- Mucopolysaccharidosis
- Chronic subdural effusions from meningitis, trauma, non-accidental injury
- Post-haemorrhagic hydrocephalus may be associated with scaphocephaly
- X-linked aqueduct stenosis
- Metabolic disease (Canavan Alexander)

Key points
- If head growth is parallel to centiles, it may be normal variant
- If progressive or symptomatic then investigate with MRI/CT or ultrasound if anterior fontanelle is open

Microcephaly

This is a physical finding not an individual disease and signs vary with causation.

Physical signs
- Head circumference <3 standard deviations
- Forehead slopes away from face
- Early closure of fontanelle is common
- Signs of associated condition or syndrome, e.g. Cornelia de Lange, cerebral malformation or craniosynostosis
- Accompanying neurological deficit may vary from mild developmental delay to severe quadriplegia
- Strabismus, cataracts or chorioretinopathy may be present
- Plot height, weight and OFC (compare with parental measurements)

Causes
- Cerebral malformations, e.g. holoprosencephaly, lissencephaly
- Congenital infections – CMV, rubella, toxoplasmosis, varicella
- Postnatal infections – encephalitis, meningitis
- Antenatal drug exposure, e.g. alcohol or phenytoin
- Hypoxic–ischaemic encephalopathy
- Inborn errors of metabolism
- First trimester intrauterine irradiation
- Trisomy 18, 13 or 21
- Familial microcephaly

Key points
- Onset at birth for primary causes and within the first 2 years of life for secondary causes
- Investigations to consider: CT/MRI, skull X-ray, TORCH screen, karyotype, metabolic screen
- Neuroimaging may demonstrate structural anomalies such as encephalomalacia, atrophy, hydrocephaly, calcification, craniosynostosis
- Prognosis depends on causation and accompanying neurological status

Moebius syndrome

Physical signs
- Bilateral facial weakness (may be asymmetrical)
- Lower face usually less affected than upper
- Mask-like expressionless face
- Bilateral abducens palsy ± other cranial nerve involvement
- Mouth constantly held open
- Swallowing difficulties – weak palate and masseter muscles
- Micrognathia
- Small tongue

Associations
- Absent pectoralis muscle
- Talipes
- Digit anomalies, e.g. brachydactyly or syndactyly
- Mental retardation in 10–15%

Key points
- Inheritance mostly sporadic but rare cases familial
- Incidence – rare
- Hypoplastic cranial nerve nuclei demonstated on MRI

Myasthenia gravis

Physical signs
- Ptosis (unilateral or bilateral)
- A variable degree of extraocular muscle weakness
- Normal pupillary response to light
- Facial weakness
    — inability to bury eyelashes
    — lack of facial expression
- Bulbar dysfunction – dysphagia, dysarthria
- Breathlessness
- Muscles demonstrate easy fatigability; however, proximal muscle weakness is variable and may improve with rest
- Tendon reflexes often normal or exaggerated but may disappear on repeated stimulation
- Look for thymectomy scar/sequelae of long-term steroid use

Associations
- Autoimmune disease, including hypothyroidism, rheumatoid arthritis, SLE and diabetes mellitus

Key points
- More common in females
- Diagnosed by tensilon test where there is improvement in symptoms following administration of cholinesterase inhibitor
- Thymomas are rare in childhood compared with adults
- Treatment – cholinergic drugs, steroids, thymectomy or plasmapheresis
- Prognosis – 90% have significant improvement or remission with treatment but this may need to be long-term

Myotonic dystrophy

Physical signs
- Characteristic facial appearance
  — myopathic facies
  — triangular mouth
  — ptosis
  — concave temples
- Frontal baldness
- Cataracts
- Peripheral weakness, especially of wrist and foot extensors
- Talipes
- Wasting of thenar and hypothenar eminences
- Myotonia (slow relaxation of muscles after contraction may be demonstrated by firm handshake or tapping the thenar eminence)
- Also shake hands with parents – one may demonstrate myotonia

Associations
- Mental retardation
- Cardiac involvement – arrhythmias, mitral valve prolapse and cardiomyopathy
- Testicular or ovarian atrophy
- Diabetes mellitus

Key points
- Autosomal dominant inheritance
- Defect is expansion of trinucleotide repeat on chromosome 19
- Often demonstrates 'anticipation', in which successive generations tend to be more severely affected
- Children with congenital myotonic dystrophy have the mother as the affected parent and present with severe hypotonia, facial weakness, feeding difficulties and contractures

Rett syndrome

Physical signs
- Psychomotor regression
- Autistic features
- Loss of purposeful hand movements
- Stereotypic activity, e.g. hand wringing or clapping
- Ataxia
- Gait apraxia
- Acquired microcephaly
- Kyphoscoliosis
- Decreased mobility
- Spastic paraparesis in advanced cases

Associations
- Epileptic seizures
- Episodic hyperventilation and periods of apnoea

Key points
- Sporadic inheritance in females
- Diagnosis based on clinical features
- Onset of disease manifestations at 6 months to 3 years
- Long-term prognosis very poor

Spina bifida

Physical signs

- Neurological signs will vary with level of lesion; 80% are lumbosacral
- High lesions may result in lower limb deformity; calipers, orthosis or a wheelchair may be required
- Tone, power, reflexes and sensation should be tested to establish levels of motor and sensory deficit
- Examine back for surgical scar, patch of hair, lipoma, skin discoloration, dermal sinus
- Hydrocephalus is commonly present due to Arnold–Chiari malformation; ventricular peritoneal shunts are often required
- Rarely, a low cranial nerve palsy results from compression of the brainstem in shallow posterior fossa by the hydrocephalus
- Kyphoscoliosis
- Strabismus may be present
- Test speech (may be 'cocktail party' in quality) and cognition
- Look for pressure sores or skin grafts to previous lesions
- Ask about/look for catheter, palpate abdomen for bladder and/or evidence of constipation (in a short case you are unlikely to be asked to examine for abnormalities of anal tone)
- Measure blood pressure

Associations

- Renal impairment due to reflux/infection
- Behavioural or emotional problems
- Precocious puberty (comment on pubertal stage in exam)
- Arnold–Chiari malformation

Key points

- Recurrence risk is approximately 5% if fist-degree relative affected
- Lesions may be detected in utero by ultrasound or raised alpha-fetoprotein
- Preconceptual folic acid supplementation reduces the risk of neural tube defects

- Lumbosacral lesions may cause poor anal tone and dribbling incontinence; thoracic lesions may cause normal anal tone but increased bladder tone, and sacral lesions may cause bladder/bowel symptoms in the absence of motor signs

Spinal muscular atrophy

ACUTE INFANTILE (WERDNIG–HOFFMANN DISEASE, SMA TYPE I)

Physical signs in infant
- Proximal weakness (progresses to quadriplegia)
- Marked hypotonia
- Areflexia
- Characteristic 'frog's leg' posture – abducted hips and flexed knees
- Alert facies
- Weak cry
- Eye movements intact
- Tongue fasciculations
- Thorax flattened laterally due to intercostal weakness
- Breathing movements cause a 'seesaw' movement of abdomen
- May have feeding tube in situ

Key points
- Autosomal recessive inheritance
- Carrier frequency 1 in 80, resulting in 1 per 25 000 births
- Gene maps to chromosome 5q12–14
- Diagnosis confirmed on electromyography
- Prognosis poor with the majority dying before 2 years

CHRONIC (KUGELBERG–WELANDER, SMA TYPE III)

Physical signs
- Older infant or child
- Waddling gait
- Slowly progressive weakness
- Wasting of proximal muscle groups
- Gower's sign positive
- Fasciculation of muscle may be present, particularly in tongue
- Calf hypertrophy occasionally present
- Absent knee jerks but preserved in ankle and upper limb

Key points

- Autosomal recessive inheritance
- Gene maps to chromosome 5q12–14
- Diagnosis made on elevated CK, typical EMG findings and muscle biopsy
- May live until adulthood

Zellweger syndrome (cerebrohepatorenal syndrome)

Physical signs (rarely older than 1 year)
- Generalised hypotonia and weakness; may show 'frog's leg' posture (abducted hips and flexed knees)
- Cataracts
- Jaundice
- High forehead
- Large anterior fontanelle
- Hypertelorism and supraorbital ridges
- Micrognathia
- Nystagmus
- Hepatomegaly

Associations
- Renal cystic dysplasia
- Intrahepatic biliary dysgenesis
- Neonatal seizures

Key points
- Autosomal recessive inheritance
- It is a peroxisomal disorder due to a defect in peroxisomal assembly and dysfunction in multiple enzyme systems
- Stippled epiphyses radiologically
- Patients usually die before 6 months of age
- Biochemical features include high levels of very long-chain fatty acids

Skin

Anhidrotic ectodermal dysplasia

Physical signs

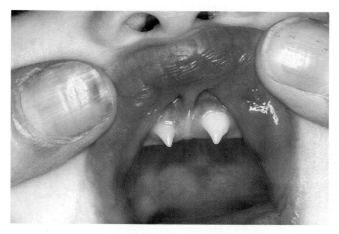

Fig. 1 Cone-shaped incisors of 3-year-old male with anhidrotic ectodermal dysplasia.

- Absent or sparse scalp hair, fine and dry; eyelashes also affected
- Smooth and finely wrinkled skin
- Cone-shaped or absent incisors (Fig. 1)
- Delayed eruption of teeth
- Saddle-shaped nose with flat nasal bridge
- Prominent forehead
- Large ears
- Thick lips
- Brittle nails with linear ridging

Key points

- Usually X-linked recessive inheritance; carrier females may show dental involvement (conical teeth)
- Absence of sweat glands makes patient susceptible to heat stroke and hyperthermia
- Approximately one-third have some degree of mental retardation
- Treatment is symptomatic, involving artificial tears to prevent corneal damage, regular dental care and prevention of overheating

Blue rubber naevus

Physical signs
- Slate grey-blue colour, raised lesion
- Usually solitary
- Occurs on limbs, lower back or buttocks

Associations
- Cavernous haemangioma of the gastrointestinal tract

Key points
- Sporadic inheritance, although some autosomal dominant familial cases have been described
- Severe gastrointestinal bleeding can occur

Clubbing

Physical signs
- Bulbous enlargement of terminal phalanx
- Loss of angle between nail bed and skin on the dorsal surface of digit
- Increased fluctuation of the nail bed
- Look for signs of the cause of the clubbing
- Check parents for clubbing if no obvious cause in patient

Causes
- Cyanotic congenital heart disease (cyanosis, thoracotomy/mediasternotomy scars)
- Infective endocarditis
- Cystic fibrosis (see p. 7)
- Bronchiectasis (see p. 5)
- Empyema
- Lung abscess
- Fibrosing alveolitis (see p. 10)
- Crohn's disease (abdominal scars)
- Ulcerative colitis (rare in childhood)
- Chronic liver disease (see p. 28)
- Hereditary

Key points
- Rarely an isolated feature; hence must search for an underlying cause

Eczema

Physical signs
- Erythematous, scaly papules on dry skin
- Chronic lichenification; thick skin with increased markings, especially around flexures
- Excoriation
- Symmetrical involvement of flexural surfaces of elbows, wrists, knees and ankles
- Pityriasis alba – hypopigmented patches on face due to chronic superficial depigmenting dermatitis
- Secondary infection may occur, causing inflammation and regional lymphadenopathy
- Signs of other atopic conditions – hay fever, asthma

Associations
- Wiskott–Aldrich syndrome (see p. 130), Jobs syndrome (see p. 124), phenylketonuria
- Secondary infections – bacterial (particularly staphylococcal) and viral
- Sleep disturbance

Key points
- Familial – 25% of families in the UK are atopic, but less than 10% develop eczema
- Usually has a chronic course but remits in 90% of children
- Herpes simplex infection may cause eczema herpeticum, which is life-threatening

Epidermolysis bullosa

A group of 16 inherited disorders characterised by a tendency to develop blisters after minimal trauma. Examples seen in examinations are likely to be *epidermolysis bullosa simplex* (EBS) or *epidermolysis bullosa dystrophica* (EBD).

Physical signs
- Bullae and blisters on hands and feet only (EBS) or over entire skin (EBD)
- Severe deformity of hands or feet (EBD only)
- Areas of hypopigmentation where bullae have ruptured
- Dystrophic or absent nails (EBD only)
- Scarring and fusion of digits, following healing of blisters (EBD only)
- Mucous membrane involvement of mouth and oesophagus (EBD only)

Associations
- Risk of malignant change in areas of scarred skin
- Oesophageal stenosis may occur in EBD due to mucosal scarring

Key points
- Autosomal dominant inheritance for EBS; EBD may be dominant or recessive
- Onset at birth for recessively inherited EBD or a few days after for other forms of EBS and EBD
- Usually improves with age
- No effective treatment; protection from trauma is essential
- High-dose prednisolone may reduce severity of bullae and mucosal involvement in infancy

Erythema nodosum

Physical signs

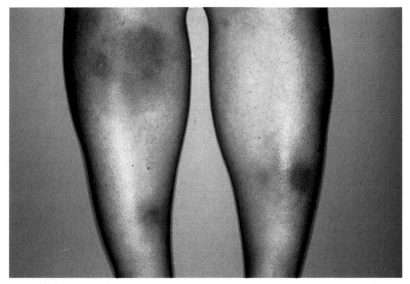

Fig. 2 Erythema nodosum.

- Tender, erythematous nodules, usually on shins (Fig. 2) but may occur on thighs or forearms
- Oedema and bruising around sites of nodules
- Swollen, painful joints
- Signs of underlying condition

Associations
- Infections – *Streptococcus*, *Mycoplasma* tuberculosis, Epstein–Barr virus
- Drugs – sulphonamides, oral contraceptive pill
- Systemic disease – inflammatory bowel disease, sarcoidosis, Behçet's disease, Hodgkin's disease

Key points

- Inflammation of subcutaneous fat (panniculitis)
- Usually resolves within 8 weeks, but persists if cause not treated
- Management involves symptomatic analgesia and treatment of the underlying condition; short courses of oral prednisolone have been used

Hypomelanosis of Ito

Physical signs
- Irregular, depigmented patches on the trunk and limbs that follow Blaschko's developmental lines
- May be unilateral or symmetrical

Assocations
- Seizures
- Mental retardation

Key points
- Sporadic inheritance with occasional autosomal dominant examples

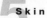

Incontinentia pigmenti

Physical signs
- Skin appearances change with time and show four stages depending on the age of the patient:
  1. *in neonates* – linear groups of blisters/vesicles on limbs and trunk
  2. *after the first few weeks* – papules with hyperkeratotic surface replace blisters
  3. bizarre, whorled slate-grey to brown macular pigmentation replaces the papules; axilla and groin affected
  4. the above fades leaving hypopigmented atrophic patches
- Eye abnormalities in 30%; microphthalmia, strabismus, cataract or optic atrophy
- Microcephaly
- Delayed dentition or absence of teeth; may have peg-shaped incisors
- Partial alopecia

Associations
- Central nervous system defects in 25%; microcephaly, epilepsy or mental retardation

Key points
- Differential diagnosis – epidermolysis bullosa (see p. 72) candidiasis, bullous impetigo, hypomelanosis of Ito (see p. 75)
- X-dominant condition – affected males die in utero; hence only seen in girls; gene for familial cases mapped to Xq28 and sporadic cases to Xp11

Klippel–Trenaunay syndrome

Physical signs
- Asymmetrical hypertrophy of one or more limbs; can involve soft tissue and bone
- Large port-wine stain on hypertrophied limb or distant skin areas
- May have polydactyly or syndactyly

Associations
- High-output cardiac failure may be found
- Vascular malformations of internal organs

Key points
- Sporadic inheritance
- Surgery may be necessary in selected cases

Molluscum contagiosum

Physical signs
- White or pink hemispherical raised lesions with central depression giving umbilicated appearance
- Multiple lesions common, up to 5–10 mm in diameter, usually in clusters
- Secondary infection can occur, with inflammation and associated regional lymphadenopathy

Associations
- Commoner in atopic and immunocompromised individuals

Key points
- Caused by a DNA poxvirus and spread by direct contact
- Benign lesions which resolve spontaneously after 6–9 months
- Cryotherapy or piercing with forceps causes inflammation and then resolution

Mongolian blue spot

Physical signs
- Grey-blue pigmented macular lesion over lumbosacral region (occasionally other areas)

Associations
- Pigmented skin types
- Down syndrome

Key points
- Benign lesion due to pigment in dermal melanocytes
- Fades during childhood

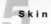

Oculocutaneous albinism

Physical signs
- White hair (sun exposure may lead to yellow tinge in tips)
- Grey or grey-blue irises
- Prominent red reflex
- Nystagmus
- Strabismus in 90%
- Decreased visual acuity (may be wearing tinted glasses or contact lenses)
- No brown pigmented lesions on skin; naevus cells produce red or purple spots due to the absence of melanin

Associations
- Cross syndrome – microphthalmia, gingival fibrosis, spasticity and mental retardation and oculocutaneous albinism
- Bleeding diasthesis in Hermansky–Pudlak syndrome
- Signs of infection and hepatosplenomegaly in Chediak–Higashi syndrome (see p. 121)

Key points
- Autosomal recessive inheritance – heterozygotes have normal pigmentation
- Can be divided into two forms by hair-bulb testing: tyrosinase negative and tyrosinase positive (more common and less severe)
- Increased incidence of skin malignancies; hence must avoid sun exposure

Port-wine stain (naevus flammeus)

Physical signs
- Macular naevus present from birth
- Colour varies from pale pink to deep purple
- Usually unilateral, involving face, trunk or limb

Associations
- Klippel–Trenaunay syndrome (see p. 77)
- Sturge–Weber syndrome (see p. 90)

Key points
- Developmental defect of mature dermal capillaries
- Present at birth and persists into middle age when darkening occurs and angiomatous nodules may develop
- Management is cosmetic using camouflage; pulsed dye laser therapy or infrared coagulation may be of value

Psoriasis

Physical signs
- Well-demarcated, raised erythematous patches with silvery scales
- Symmetrical plaques commonly on extensor surfaces of knees and elbows; other sites include scalp, sacrum and sites of trauma/scars (Koebner phenomenon)
- Yellow-brown pustules (sterile) may occur on palms and soles in the absence of other skin signs
- Nail changes include pitting, subungual hyperkeratosis, onycholysis (lifting of the nail plate distally), yellow 'salmon' patches, splinter haemorrhages

Associations
- Psoriatic arthropathy (in 5% of cases) – commonly affects distal interphalangeal joints and sacroiliac joints, although any large and small joints may be involved
- Napkin psoriasis – rash resembling candidiasis spreading outside nappy area. Resolves quickly but there is an increased risk of psoriasis in later life
- Guttate psoriasis – multiple pale red plaques <1 cm in diameter ('raindrop' lesions) on trunk and limbs following streptococcal sore throat; resolves spontaneously or turns to plaque psoriasis in later life

Key points
- 10% of psoriatics present before 4 years of age; 30% before 20 years
- Affects 2% of white populations in temperate climates: rare in pigmented skins
- HLA antigens B13, B17, CW6, DR7 and B27 are associated
- Differential diagnosis includes pityriasis rosea; may resemble guttate psoriasis although herald patch precedes it and the oval lesions usually run along rib lines
- Aetiology unknown but the characteristic feature is rapid epidermal turnover time
- Treatment is usually with topical dithranol tar preparations; systemic therapy is rarely required

Strawberry naevus (capillary haemangioma)

Physical sign
- Raised, well-demarcated, compressible lesion with a bright red surface

Associations
- Kasabach–Merritt syndrome: strawberry naevus associated with platelet sequestration, thrombocytopenia and haemorrhage
- Cardiac failure, feeding or visual difficulties may occur with large lesions
- Bleeding may follow trauma

Key points
- Common lesion present in 10% of infants < 1 year; most frequently on head and neck
- Lesion results from benign angioplastic proliferation
- Appears within a few weeks of birth and enlarges over first 6 months of life
- Spontaneous regression follows with the surface initially becoming white
- Complete regression in 50% by 5 years and 90% by 9 years of age
- High-dose steroids are indicated to treat Kasabach–Merritt or if feeding or vision impaired

Neurocutaneous

McCune–Albright syndrome (polyostotic fibrous dysplasia)

Physical signs
- Precocious puberty (commoner in girls than boys)
- Café-au-lait spots with characteristic ragged edges
- Evidence of fractures, due to thinning and sclerosis of bones
- Skeletal asymmetry due to polyostotic fibrous dysplasia
- Abdominal scar following adrenalectomy (for adrenal hyperplasia/Cushing's syndrome)

Associations
- Multiple endocrinopathies with hyperfunction (thyroid, parathyroid, adrenals, growth hormone)

Key points
- Non-familial inheritance
- Average age of onset of precocious puberty is about 3–4 years
- Abnormal activation of cyclic AMP regulation of endocrine glands occurs
- No effective treatment for suppression of endocrine dysfunction available
- Asymptomatic bone lesions require no therapy

Neurofibromatosis

Two distinct forms of neurofibromatosis exist: type 1 and type 2. Separate genes are responsible for these two forms, although both result from abnormal neural crest differentiation.

TYPE 1

Physical signs

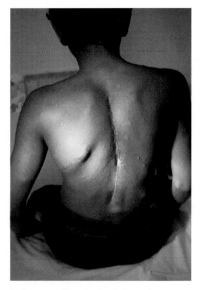

Fig. 3 Café-au-lait spots in neurofibromatosis type 1.

Two or more of the following are needed to make the diagnosis:

- five or more café-au-lait spots greater than 5 mm in diameter pre-puberty (Fig. 3) or 15 mm post-puberty; present in almost all cases
- axillary or inguinal freckling – hyperpigmented spots ~ 3 mm in diameter
- two or more Lisch nodules – hamartomas of the iris (often only discovered on slit-lamp examination)

- two or more *neurofibromas* or one *plexiform neurofibroma*. Neurofibromas are soft, firm, rubbery subcutaneous lesions which classically involve the skin but may be found along peripheral nerves or blood vessels. Plexiform neurofibromas result from thickening of nerve trunks leading to tissue overgrowth. Commonly found in the orbital or temporal regions, they are associated with hyperpigmentation of overlying skin
- bony lesions – include scoliosis, kyphoscoliosis, pseudarthrosis of the tibia
- optic glioma, usually asymptomatic but may cause visual disturbance; afferent pupillary defects may be found
- first-degree relative with neurofibromatosis type 1.

Associations
- Mental retardation
- Seizures: complex–partial and tonic–clonic
- Hypertension
- Neurofibrosarcoma arising in a neurofibroma
- Congenital buphthalmos (see p. 95)

Key points
- 90% of cases of neurofibromatosis are type 1
- Autosomal dominant inheritance with high penetrance but variable expression
- Gene located on chromosome 17q22
- Wilms' tumours and phaeochromocytomas occur more commonly than in the general population
- Management includes genetic counselling and treatment of complications

TYPE 2

Physical signs
One of the following is needed to make a diagnosis:

- bilateral eighth cranial nerve tumours on neuroimaging consistent with acoustic neuromas. Acoustic neuromas may lead to hearing loss, facial weakness, dizziness and unsteadiness

- first-degree relative with neurofibromatosis type 2 and either eighth nerve masses or any two of the following: neurofibroma, schwannoma, glioma, meningioma or posterior subscapular lenticular opacities.

Associations
- Café-au-lait spots and neurofibromas
- Central nervous system tumours, including gliomas, schwannomas and meningiomas

Key points
- Account for 10% of cases of neurofibromatosis
- Autosomal dominant inheritance; gene located on chromosome 22q
- Signs of acoustic neuromas often not present until second or third decade
- Management includes genetic counselling and treatment of acoustic neuromas and other tumours

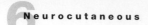

Sturge–Weber syndrome

Physical signs
- Port-wine stain – flat red vascular naevus within the cutaneous distribution of ophthalmic and/or maxillary divisions of the trigeminal nerve
- Ipsilateral exophthalmos, colobomata, buphthalmos or glaucoma
- Contralateral hemiparesis (in 30%)
- Homonymous hemianopic field deficit (common)
- Telangiectasia of conjunctiva
- Fundus may be dark red and the retina may be detached

Associations
- Ipsilateral leptomeningeal angiomatosis and intracranial calcification
- Epilepsy
- Mental retardation

Key points
- Usually sporadic
- Incidence – port-wine stain, 1 in 5000; Sturge–Weber syndrome, 1 in 30 000
- Ophthalmic complications only occur if the port-wine stain involves the ophthalmic division of the trigeminal nerve
- Characteristic changes seen on CT scan and skull X-rays (tram-lining)
- Progressive hemiplegia, mental retardation and deterioration in seizure control can occur

Tuberous sclerosis

Physical signs

Fig. 4 'Ash leaf' spot in tuberous sclerosis.

- Amelanotic naevi (ash leaf spots) (Fig. 4); may need Wood's light to see
- Adenoma sebaceum – erythematous papular acneiform rash over nose and cheeks (rare under 2 years of age, seen in 50% by 5 years and 100% by 35 years of age)
- Shagreen patch – raised irregular rough area usually over the lumbar region
- Subungual fibroma – fleshy outgrowth of nail bed of fingers or toes (rare in childhood)
- Gingival fibromas
- Café-au-lait patches (in 5% of cases)
- Learning difficulties and developmental delay
- Palpable kidneys, due to renal angiomyolipomata or polycystic kidneys
- Retinal phakomata – raised mushroom-like lesion near optic disc
- Parents may have stigmata of disease

Associations
- Epilepsy in 95%
- Mental retardation in 50%
- Intracranial calcification in 50%
- Cardiac rhabdomyomata (usually asymptomatic with no signs)

Key points
- Autosomal dominant inheritance; about half the cases are sporadic due to new mutations
- Incidence ~ 1 in 50 000
- Gene located on chromosome 9q34
- May present with infantile spasms
- 80% have renal involvement
- Multiple intracranial gliotic hamartomas and nodules may undergo malignant change

Eyes

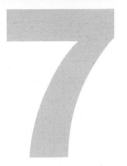

Aniridia

Physical signs
- Absent irises, usually bilateral
- Photophobia
- Impaired visual acuity
- Lens opacities and macular hyperplasia
- Nephrectomy scars if a Wilms' tumour removed
- Hypertension (if genitourinary anomalies)

Associations
- Ataxia + aniridia = Gillespie syndrome (autosomal recessive)
- Wilms' tumour, genitourinary anomalies and mental retardation associated with deletion on short arm of chromosome 11
- Buphthalmos

Key points
- Due to failure of mesoderm to grow from the root of the iris
- Sporadic or autosomal dominant inheritance
- Children with aniridia should be checked for chromosome 11 deletion as this carries increased risk of Wilms' tumours

Buphthalmos (congenital glaucoma)

Physical signs
- Hazy or cloudy cornea, due to corneal oedema
- Blepharospasm (eyelid squeezing)
- Photophobia
- Reduced or absent red reflex
- Epiphoria (tearing)
- Enlarged orbital globe
- Cupping of optic disc and optic atrophy
- Decreased visual acuity and blindness if untreated

Associations
- Stickler–Marshall syndrome: mid-face hypoplasia, epicanthic folds, stiff joints (autosomal dominant)
- Sturge–Weber syndrome
- Neurofibromatosis
- Congenital rubella syndrome
- Marfan syndrome
- Other ocular abnormalities such as aniridia, cataract, ectopia lentis

Key points
- Sporadic cases or inheritance may be autosomal dominant or recessive
- 4–5% recurrence risk for offspring and siblings of isolated cases
- Incidence – 1 in 12 500 births
- Management involves urgent surgical assessment and intervention

Cataract

Physical signs
- Opacity within the lens – ranges from complete opacification (white lens) to specks of calcification
- Loss of red reflex if mature cataract
- Unilateral or bilateral
- Reduced visual acuity may occur and be accompanied by nystagmus and signs of underlying problems or syndromes

Associations
- Chromosomal disorders – trisomy 13, 18 and 21 and Turner syndromes
- Congenital infections – toxoplasmosis, herpes simplex, rubella, cytomegalovirus
- Metabolic disorders – galactosaemia, diabetes mellitus, hypoparathyroidism, mucopolysaccharidoses, Lowe syndrome, Zellweger syndrome, Wilson disease
- Drugs – steroids
- Miscellaneous – myotonic dystrophy, osteogenesis imperfecta, Apert and Crouzon syndromes, Alport syndrome, congenital ichthyosis, incontinentia pigmenti, trauma

Key points
- 10% are hereditary (autosomal dominant, recessive or X-linked recessive)
- Potential for good vision following cataract surgery is related to age at which opacity developed and length of time present
- Early treatment of galactosaemia may reverse lens opacities

Coloboma

Physical signs
- Developmental defect in some portion of the eye
- Usually inferior and nasal
- Any ocular structure may be involved (eyelid, iris, lens, retina)

Associations
- CHARGE association
- Goldenhar syndrome (see p. 160)
- Treacher–Collins syndrome (see p. 173)

Key points
- Results from failure of fusion of the choroidal fissure in development
- Iris usually involved but may extend into ciliary body, retina, choroid and optic nerve
- Isolated coloboma may be inherited as an autosomal dominant trait
- Management is determined by site and size of defect

Heterochromia

Physical sign
● Asymmetry in the colour of the iris

Associations
● Waardenburg syndrome – heterochromia, white hair in forelock, sensorineural deafness, autosomal dominant inheritance
● Congenital Horner syndrome (the eye with Horner's is lighter in colour)
● Secondary to inflammation or trauma to eye
● Wilms' tumour or cervicothoracic neuroblastoma

Key points
● Usually sporadic, occasionally autosomal dominant

Microphthalmos

Physical sign
- Reduction in size of all ocular structures

Associations
- Cat's eye syndrome – uveal coloboma, renal malformations, imperforate anus
- CHARGE syndrome
- Congenital infections – cytomegalovirus, rubella and toxoplasmosis
- Goldenhar syndrome (see p. 160)

Key points
- Microphthalmia associated with colobomata is usually an autosomal dominant inheritance
- Recurrence risk in siblings of isolated cases is 10%
- May be secondary to ocular disease or inflammation

Optic atrophy

Physical signs
- Pale, clearly delineated optic discs
- Yellow/grey discs with blurred margins if atrophy is secondary to papilloedema
- Paucity and attenuation of retinal vessels crossing the optic discs
- Enlargement of optic cup with visible lamina cribrosa giving 'pinhole' appearance
- Consensual reaction of pupil to light but no direct reaction
- Decreased visual acuity
- Visual field defects, including central scotoma

Associations
- DIDMOAD (diabetes insipidus + diabetes mellitus + optic atrophy + deafness)
- Intracranial tumours, including those in and around the pituitary and optic nerve gliomas
- Benign intracranial hypertension
- Friedreich ataxia
- Post-inflammatory from optic neuritis
- Neurodegenerative syndromes and inborn errors of metabolism

Key points
- In autosomal recessive forms, earlier onset of visual loss
- Leber optic atrophy (male: female ratio = 6:1); bilateral involvement in early adolescence with retinal oedema and normal retinal vessels

Papilloedema

Physical signs

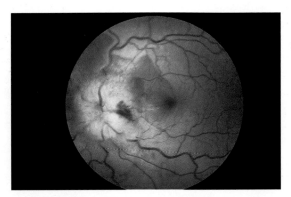

Fig. 5   Blurring of optic disc margins in papilloedema.

- Blurring of the disc margins (may be asymmetric) (Fig. 5)
- Optic cup obliterated
- Hyperaemic discs due to superficial capillaries
- Intra-retinal exudates and haemorrhages
- Normal visual acuity, unless haemorrhages involve macula
- Normal pupillary reflexes

Associations
- Intracranial space-occupying lesions (tumour, abscess, haematoma)
- Hydrocephalus
- Foster–Kennedy syndrome: optic atrophy due to frontal lobe tumour pressing on optic nerve and contralateral papilloedema secondary to raised intracranial pressure
- Benign intracranial hypertension

Key points
- Swollen optic disc can occur in hypertension or optic neuritis
- Conditions mimicking papilloedema include drusen, myelinated nerve fibre glial abnormalities
- Papilloedema needs urgent investigation with neuroimaging
- Prolonged papilloedema can result in the development of optic atrophy (see p. 100)

Retinitis pigmentosa

Physical signs (Fig. 6)

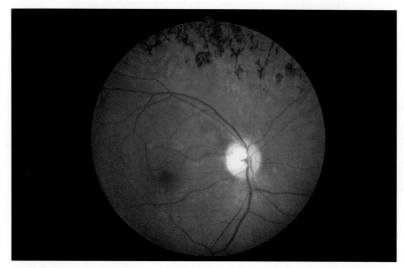

Fig. 6 Retinitis pigmentosa.

- Early stages – clumps of pigment in peripheral retina, arteriolar narrowing, optic disc pallor
- Pigment deposition in peripheral part of retina giving classical 'bone corpuscle' pattern advances progressively towards central retina
- Tunnel vision followed by loss of central vision as disease progresses

Associations
- Usher syndrome – deafness and retinitis pigmentosa (autosomal recessive inheritance)
- Refsum syndrome – neuropathy, ataxia, deafness, ichthyosis (autosomal recessive inheritance)
- Laurence–Moon–Biedl syndrome
- Abetalipoproteinaemia – acanthocytes, ataxia and lipoprotein abnormalities
- Renal diseases – Fanconi syndrome, cystinosis, cystinuria, oxalosis

Key points

- Can present with poor night vision
- Inheritance is autosomal recessive (50%), dominant or X-linked recessive
- Carrier females of the X-linked recessive form may be identified by fundoscopy and electroretinography
- Other causes of pigmented retina include congenital infection, metabolic disorders (e.g. cystinosis) and drugs

Retinoblastoma

Physical signs
- Leucocoria (white pupil)
- Loss of red reflex
- Elevated yellow or white tumour mass with dilated retinal vessels on fundoscopy
- Multiple tumour deposits may be present in each eye
- Prosthetic eye
- Visual field and acuity defects, depending on site and size of tumour deposits

Key points
- Deletion of part of long arm of chromosome 13 predisposes to retinoblastoma
- One third are bilateral
- 50% risk to offspring if bilaterally affected and 5–10% if unilateral involvement
- 2–3% risk to siblings if bilateral involvement and 1% if unilateral disease
- Treatment involves enucleation and chemotherapy. Radio therapy avoided if possible as high risk of second tumour in radiation field
- Greater than 90% survival in non-hereditary forms, which have high risk of second malignancies (bone tumours)

Musculoskeletal

Achondroplasia

Physical signs
- Disproportionately large head
- Prominent forehead, small face, depressed nasal bridge and relatively prominent jaw
- Small stature (usual length at birth is 46–48 cm; average adult height is 124 cm for women and 131 cm for men)
- Rhizomelic limb shortening – proximal segments of limbs relatively short
- Short, broad hands and feet; lack of full adduction of fingers in extension, giving rise to the typical trident hand
- Lumbar lordosis, thoracolumbar kyphosis and protuberant abdomen
- Bowed legs with internal tibial torsion and waddling gait

Associations
- Neurological complications – hydrocephalus, spinal cord compression at the foramen magnum
- Obstructive sleep apnoea
- Recurrent otitis media, conductive or sensorineural deafness

Key points
- Autosomal dominant inheritance; however, 80% of cases represent fresh mutation
- The most common skeletal dysplasia with a frequency of 1 in 20 000 births
- Results from decreased rate of endochondral bone formation with normal membranous bone formation and articular cartilage
- No specific treatment available, but surgical intervention for hydrocephalus or spinal cord compression may be required
- For the heterozygous individual, there is a normal life expectancy if serious complications are avoided

Ankylosing spondylitis

Physical signs
- Limitation of motion of lumbar spine in anterior flexion, lateral flexion and extension
- Flattening of the normal lumbar lordosis and accentuated dorsal kyphosis
- Restricted chest expansion
- Neck in flexed position giving rise to a stooped position
- Check for arthritis, particularly in the hip or knee

Associations
- Association with HLA-B27 allele
- Episodes of anterior uveitis in 25% of patients

Key points
- Rare in early childhood; clinical features usually appear in second or third decade
- Commoner in boys
- Probably an autoimmune response resulting from interaction in a susceptible individual with infectious agents, e.g. *Klebsiella*, *Yersinia*
- Inflammatory lesions affect cartilage, subchondral bone and periosteum; tendon and fascia insertion sites often affected (enthesopathy)
- Characteristic X-ray changes – sacroiliac joints become fused; spinal apophyseal, facet and costovertebral joints show bony fusion

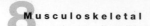

Cleidocranial dysplasia

Physical signs
- Large cranium with delayed closure of fontanelles and sutures
- Brachycephaly
- Frontal and parietal bossing and a supraglabellar depression
- Hypoplasia of the maxilla
- Depressed broadened nasal bridge
- High arched palate with or without a cleft
- Delayed dentition
- Narrow upper thorax and drooping shoulders
- Partial or complete aplasia of the clavicles, allowing hypermobility of the shoulders
- Narrow pelvis and small stature
- Long second metacarpals and tapering distal phalanges

Associations
- Syringomyelia

Key points
- Autosomal dominant inheritance but with a variable expression; approximately one-third appear to be new mutations
- Radiologically numerous wormian bones and delayed ossification, especially of pubic bones
- Normal life expectancy and intelligence
- Early dental/orthodontic care is usually indicated

Ehlers–Danlos syndrome

Physical signs
- Marked skin hyperelasticity
- Increased skin fragility – slow healing leaves 'cigarette paper'-like scars, particularly over the forehead, knees and elbows
- Very elastic and pliable ears
- Easy bruising – check for evidence of skin and soft tissue haemorrhages
- Molluscoid pseudotumours and spheroids over knees, shins and elbows
- Hypermobility of joints
- Musculoskeletal deformities may occur, e.g. kyphoscoliosis, pes planus
- Varicose veins commonly occur

Associations
- At least nine different types have been defined (based on clinical, genetic and biochemical findings) with variable findings

Key points
- Heterogeneous group of disorders resulting from defective connective tissue, most likely collagen abnormality
- Pattern of inheritance varies depending on type
- Type 1 (gravis type) most commonly described; autosomal dominant inheritance
- No specific treatment; avoiding trauma and unnecessary surgery is important

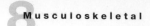

Juvenile chronic arthritis

This term encompasses a heterogeneous group of disorders. Classification is based on clinical features at presentation and disease progression and helps structure an approach: systemic arthritis, oligoarthritis, polyarticular arthritis (rheumatoid-factor positive or negative), enthesitis arthritis, psoriatic arthritis or unclassified. Be prepared to demonstrate appropriate joint assessment and awareness of relevant extra-articular features.

Physical signs

Joints
Look, feel, move (active then passive) joints in a systematic may. Actively involved joints.

- swollen with periarticular thickening or joint effusion
- warm and tender to touch
- limited joint movement; painful to move

Extra-articular features
Features found depend on the type of JCA. The following list outlines the range:

- General: comment on general appearance and growth
- Skin: nail pitting and psoriatic rash; fine red-pink maculopapular rash; nodules
- Eyes: iridocyclitis (detected on slit lamp examination) may lead to posterior synechiae causing irregular shaped pupil cataract
- Systemic examination: cardiomegaly, pericardits, pleuritis, hepatosplenomegaly, lymphadenopathy
- Limbs. Observe for and comment on: chronic joint deformity; muscle bulk and power; gait

Key points
- Annual incidence rates in UK 10 per 100 000
- Systemic arthritis (11%) usually presents in 1–4 years age group with high spiking fever, intermittent rash and polyarticular arthritis
- Oligoarthritis (four or less joints) affects mainly young girls (peak age 3 years); (active then passive) joints in a systematic way.

Klippel–Feil anomaly

Physical signs
- Short webbed neck
- Limitation of head and neck movements, particularly side-to-side and rotational movements
- Low posterior hairline

Associations
- Other bony abnormalities such as scoliosis, cervical ribs and Sprengel shoulder (see Sprengel deformity)
- Urinary tract anomalies such as horseshoe kidney, unilateral renal agenesis
- Ocular defects in ~ 20% of cases, e.g. squint, ptosis, nystagmus
- Cardiac abnormalities, particularly ventricular septal defect
- Cleft palate

Key points
- The constant finding is congenital fusion of the cervical vertebrae
- Incidence of 1 in 40 000 live births with a female to male ratio of 3:2
- Most cases are sporadic although occurrence in some families points to autosomal dominant and autosomal recessive patterns of inheritance
- Most important complication is cervical cord injury as a consequence of occipitocervical instability
- Normal life span expected if there are no serious associated abnormalities or complications

Osteogenesis imperfecta

Physical signs
There are four major types (see below); type 1 is the most common and has the following features:

- blue-grey sclerae
- fragile bones prone to fractures, particularly arms and legs
- bowing deformity of long bones
- hypermobility of joints, especially small joints of hands and feet
- kyphosis – usually mild and occurring in later life
- teeth in type IA – normal
- teeth in type IB – opalescent, often a yellow-brown colour and easily cracked or worn
- hearing often impaired (usually conductive but can be mixed or sensory)
- tendency to easy bruising.

Associations
- X-rays show wormian bones in skull and generalised osteopenia
- Aortic regurgitation and mitral valve prolapse may occur
- Tendon sprains and avulsions occur

Key points
- Type I inherited as autosomal dominant; biochemically there is a defect in the production of type I procollagen
- 10% have fractures at birth and the majority before 5 years of age; management is largely supportive and most have a normal life span
- Type II – extreme fragility with intrauterine fractures; often stillborn or early neonatal death
- Type III – autosomal recessive; initial blue sclerae gradually fade; progressive limb and chest deformity; high mortality in third and fourth decades from cardiorespiratory failure
- Type IV – autosomal dominant with normal sclerae and similar bone disease to type I

Poland anomaly

Physical signs
- Unilateral hand malformation
  - syndactyly – either partial or complete, usually involving the soft tissues; frequently the index and middle fingers are affected
  - short digits – phalanges, most often the middle ones, short or absent
- Ipsilateral aplasia or hypoplasia of the sternal head of pectoralis major
- Ipsilateral aplasia of breast tissue

Associations
- Other reported findings include hemivertebrae, hypoplasia of upper ribs, renal anomalies, Sprengel deformity (see p. 114)
- Association with Moebius syndrome (see p. 57)

Key points
- Most cases are sporadic
- Three times more common in males
- 75% right-handed
- Normal life expectancy

Sprengel deformity

Physical signs
- Elevated scapula (a normal scapula is usually between T2 and T7 levels)
- Small scapula lying closer to midline
- Limitation in movement in ipsilateral arm

Associations
- Other skeletal anomalies, e.g. hemivertebrae, fused vertebrae, chest deformities
- Poland syndrome (see p. 113)
- Often a communication of tissue between scapula and vertebrae

Key points
- Most cases are sporadic although autosomal dominant inheritance has been reported
- In severe cases, reconstructive surgery can improve function and appearance

Systemic lupus erythematosus (SLE)

Physical signs

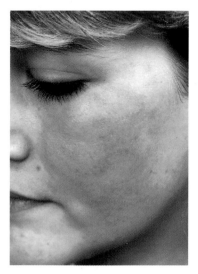

Fig. 7 Erythema in SLE.

- Skin – various rashes seen, including erythematous rash (Fig. 7) over malar eminences ('butterfly rash'), maculopapular rashes, photosensitivity rashes, telangiectasia and purpuric lesions
- Patchy alopecia
- Oral and nasopharyngeal ulcers, usually painless
- Arthritis and/or arthralgia is often symmetrical and commonly occurs in proximal interphalangeal, metacarpophalangeal, knee and wrist joints
- Respiratory involvement may include pleurisy (check for 'rub') and pleural effusion
- Pericarditis – check for evidence of pericardial rub
- Hypertension
- Central nervous involvement may result in cognitive impairment, cranial nerve palsy, chorea, ataxia

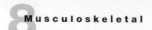

Associations
- Renal involvement is extremely common – check urine for haematuria ± proteinuria, measure blood pressure
- Haematological abnormalities are common and include haemolytic anaemia, leucopenia, thrombocytopenia
- Constitutional symptoms are common at presentation and during exacerbation, e.g. fever, weight loss, fatigue
- Cardiac involvement – myocarditis, endocarditis (Libman–Sachs)

Key points
- Peak incidence in childhood is 11–15 years, with a female preponderance (female: male = 8:1)
- Autoimmune disease of inflammation and vasculitis involving many systems
- Various autoantibody associations: antinuclear antibody-positive in most cases but anti-dsDNA and anti-Smith more specific
- Drug therapies used – antimalarials, NSAIDs, steroids, azathioprine, cyclophosphamide
- Immunosuppression and renal failure are the major causes of mortality and morbidity, but overall 10-year survival rate is now > 85%

Thrombocytopenia – absent radius (TAR) syndrome

Physical signs
- Bilateral absence of the radius
- Radial deviation of hands
- Hypoplasia of carpals and phalanges
- Thumbs *always* present (c.f. Fanconi's anaemia; see p. 122)
- Hypoplasia of humerus (often present)
- Inspect for purpura

Associations
- Cardiac anomalies such as atrial septal defect or tetralogy of Fallot are present in 30%
- Short stature is common
- Lower limb deformities
- Allergy to cow's milk often noted

Key points
- Autosomal recessive inheritance
- 90% have symptoms related to thrombocytopenia (e.g. purpura, nosebleeds, bloody stools) in the first 4 months
- Platelet counts, often $15–30 \times 10^9/L$ in infancy, tend to improve towards normal range by adulthood
- Thrombocytopenia is fluctuating and often aggravated by intercurrent infections and stress
- Significant mortality in first year of life largely related to intracranial bleeding
- Treatment largely supportive

Haematology / immunology

9

Bloom syndrome

Physical signs
- Short stature
- Bird-like fine featured facies with small head
- Prominent ears
- High arched palate
- Telangiectatic erythematous lesions of face in malar distribution and on eyelids; may also occur on ears, arms and hands
- Photosensitivity
- Café-au-lait spots in 50%
- Toe syndactyly, or absent toes
- Supernumary digits and/or clinodactyly
- Hypospadias
- Cryptorchidism

Associations
- Leukaemia and other malignancies including squamous cell carcinoma

Key points
- Autosomal recessive inheritance, more common in Ashkenazi Jews
- Male:female = 1.5:1
- Rare chromosome breakage syndrome
- Feeding difficulties may occur in infancy
- Differential diagnosis – Fanconi anaemia (but no learning difficulties in Bloom syndrome)

Chediak–Higashi syndrome

Physical signs
- Hypopigmentation of eyes, skin and hair (may be grey)
- Generalised lymphadenopathy (accelerated phase in second and third decades)
- Gingivitis
- Hepatosplenomegaly
- Cranial nerve deficits, including nystagmus and bitemporal hemianopia
- Muscle weakness
- Ataxia
- Decreased tendon reflexes
- Peripheral sensory loss
- Learning difficulties and developmental delay

Associations
- Recurrent severe bacterial infections and a mild bleeding diasthesis occur

Key points
- Rare
- Autosomal recessive inheritance
- Unknown molecular defect leading to abnormal granule morphogenesis
- Diagnosed on finding giant lysosomal granules in blood or bone marrow myeloid cells
- Majority die of infections or in 'accelerated phase' in second or third decade

Fanconi anaemia

Physical signs
- Short stature
- Epicanthic folds, hypertelorism, broad nasal bridge, low-set ears and micrognathia
- Microcephaly, flat head, frontal bossing, sloped forehead
- Choanal atresia
- Strabismus, nystagmus, ptosis, cataracts, small iris
- Generalised hyperpigmentation (trunk and neck), café-au-lait or hypopigmented patches
- Abnormal thumbs – absent, rudimentary or bifid
- Absent or abnormal radii (only with abnormal thumbs)
- Clinodactyly, polydactyly, enlarged or short fingers
- Hypogenitalia, undescended testes, micropenis, phimosis, abnormal urethra
- Umbilical hernia
- Scars may be present from oesophageal, jejunal or duodenal atresia repairs
- Ectopic kidneys, renal masses due to hydronephrosis
- Spina bifida, sacrococcygeal sinus, scoliosis
- Sprengel deformity (see p. 114)
- Learning difficulties and developmental delay

Associations
- Cardiac anomalies including ventricular septal defect, patent ductus arteriosus, peripheral pulmonary stenosis
- Greater than 15% develop malignancy; 50% are myeloid leukaemia; liver tumours common

Key points
- Autosomal recessive inheritance, gene frequency = 1 in 300
- Diagnosis made by chromosome breakage studies
- 50% respond to androgens, although relapse occurs when they are discontinued
- Bone marrow transplantation may offer cure

- Predicted life expectancy is 16 years of age
- Differential diagnosis – Bloom syndrome; distinguished from thrombocytopenia and absent radius by the presence of abnormal thumbs

Job syndrome (Hyperimmunoglobulin E syndrome)

Physical signs
- Short stature
- Coarse facies with broad nasal bridge and prominent nose
- Craniosynostosis (rare)
- Red hair and fair skin
- Hyperextensible joints
- 'Cold' cutaneous skin abscesses, especially of head and neck
- Scarring from recurrent staphylococcal skin infections, abscesses and impetigo
- Chronic eczema-like dermatitis
- Mucocutaneous candidiasis with dystrophic finger- and toenail changes
- Keratoconjunctivitis
- Glue ear and chronic ear and sinus infections
- Thoracotomy scars following lung cyst resection

Associations
- Recurrent staphylococcal infections of skin and lower respiratory tract

Key points
- Diagnosed by serum IgE >2500 IU/ml and peripheral blood eosinophilia
- Autosomal dominant inheritance with variable penetrance
- Management involves prophylactic anti-staphylococcal antibiotics and aggressive treatment of infections
- Differential diagnosis – atopic dermatitis, Wiskott–Aldrich syndrome, chronic granulomatous disease
- Experimental treatments include gamma interferon and plasmapheresis
- Prognosis is good with aggressive management; small risk of developing lymphoid malignancies

Purpura

Petechiae (<2 mm), purpura (2–10 mm) and echymoses (>10 mm) do not blanch on pressure. Important causes of purpura unlikely to be seen in the exam include acute meningococcaemia, disseminated intravascular coagulopathy (DIC), whooping cough and pancytopenia. More likely causes will be Wiskott–Aldrich syndrome (see p. 130), Henoch–Schönlein purpura, idiopathic thrombocytopenic purpura, thrombocytopenia and absent radius (TAR) syndrome (see p. 117), Bernard–Soulier syndrome or Kassabach–Merritt syndrome.

HENOCH–SCHÖNLEIN PURPURA

Physical signs
- Erythematous maculopapular purpuric rash with petechiae, most commonly on buttocks and extensor surfaces of legs and elbows
- Localised oedema, and excoriations from itching
- Painful joint swelling
- No lymphadenopathy nor hepatosplenomegaly

Associations
- Usually follows an acute infection

Key points
- Normal platelet count
- Immune complex, type III hypersensitivity reaction
- Self-limiting in majority of cases
- Intussusception and renal failure are rare complications

IDIOPATHIC THROMBOCYTOPENIC PURPURA (ITP)

Physical signs
- Bruises or purpuric rash anywhere on body
- Petechial haemorrhages
- Mucosal bleeding (uncommon but important)
- Retinal haemorrhages (uncommon but important)
- No lymphadenopathy nor hepatosplenomegaly
- Gastrointestinal bleeding and haematuria are uncommon

Associations
- ~75% have preceding viral infection in the 2 weeks prior to onset

Key points
- Platelet count $< 50 \times 10^9/L$
- Immune complex formation and complement deposition on platelets may be the explanation
- 90% recover spontaneously within 6 months
- Management may include steroids or immunoglobulins
- Bone marrow examination should be performed prior to administration of steroids
- Splenectomy may be indicated for chronic ITP
- Differential diagnoses include any cause of bone marrow infiltration

Sickle cell anaemia

Cases may have no physical manifestations or multisystem involvement.

Physical signs
- Pallor and signs of anaemia or jaundice
- Overgrowth of anterior maxilla with cosmetic or dental problems
- Delayed growth and sexual maturity
- Central venous access (if on transfusion programme)
- Joint swelling and/or effusions, or chronic joint disease
- Leg ulcers, especially around ankles, are rare in the first decade but commoner with advancing years
- Aseptic necrosis of femoral heads causing limp or necessitating hip replacement
- Short digits secondary to dactylitis (unlikely to see acute episode in exams)
- Hepatomegaly
- Splenomegaly – repeated splenic infarction leads to a small fibrotic non-palpable spleen
- Ejection systolic murmur or signs of cardiac failure due to anaemia
- Evidence of cerebrovascular accidents including hemiplegia
- Visual field defects (due to cerebral infarction)
- Proliferative retinopathy and/or retinal haemorrhages

Associations
- Overwhelming sepsis with *Streptococcus pneumoniae*, *Haemophilus* and *Meningococcus*
- Splenic sequestration, aplastic and vaso-occlusive crises

Key points
- Autosomal recessive inheritance
- Replacement of glutamic acid with valine at position 6 on the beta-globin chain

- Diagnosis made by haemoglobin electrophoresis
- Management includes regular folic acid, prophylactic penicillin, vaccination (pneumococcal and HIb), transfusion programmes and psychosocial support
- Bone marrow transplantation offers the only cure

Thalassaemia

Thalassaemias encompass a heterogenous group of anaemias of varying severity. The clinical features outlined below are for homozygous β-thalassaemia

Physical signs
- Frontal bossing, maxillary overgrowth, epicanthic folds and broad nasal bridge
- Anaemia, jaundice (secondary to haemolysis) or skin pigmentation (from iron and melanin deposition)
- Short stature and delayed puberty
- Periungual and palmar crease pigmentation
- Signs of chronic liver disease
- Cardiomyopathy, congestive cardiac failure, murmurs (due to anaemia)
- Desferrioxamine injection sites
- Hepatosplenomegaly and ascites
- Splenectomy scar may be present
- Peripheral oedema secondary to liver disease or congestive cardiac failure
- Cataracts and retinopathy (due to desferrioxamine therapy)

Associations
- Hypothyroidism, hypoparathyroidism and diabetes mellitus may develop due to iron overload

Key points
- Group of disorders with imbalanced production of one of the globin lines and hypochromic, microcytic anaemia
- Diagnosis made on haemoglobin electrophoresis
- Autosomal recessive inheritance; heterozygote carriers are usually asymptomatic
- Blood transfusions and iron chelation form mainstay of management

Wiskott–Aldrich syndrome

Physical signs
- Male
- Bruises, petechiae and purpura due to thrombocytopenia
- Eczema, may be infected
- Scarring from previous pyogenic infections (skin and chest)
- Central venous access (e.g. portacath or Hickman line)
- Splenectomy scar may be present
- Hepatosplenomegaly, lymphadenopathy
- Rhinorrhoea and glue ear

Associations
- More than 10% develop malignancies – leukaemia or lymphomas (commonly extranodal, e.g. brain)
- Eosinophilia and elevated immunoglobulin E

Key points
- X-linked inheritance; gene located at Xp11.2
- Immunodeficiency results from both humoral and cellular deficiencies
- May present in infancy with gastrointestinal bleeding or following circumcision
- Splenectomy improves the low platelet count but increases risk of sepsis with encapsulated organisms
- Management includes immunoglobulin infusions to reduce incidence of infections, irradiated platelet infusions and aggressive antibiotic therapy
- HLA-matched bone marrow transplantation is the treatment of choice

Metabolic and endocrine

Diabetes mellitus

Long-standing insulin-dependent diabetes mellitus with neurovascular complications can produce a variety of physical signs. Although signs are less common than in adults, they are still important and the candidate should be aware of the range of possible findings.

Physical signs
- Poor growth
- Hands – fingertip prick marks (from blood glucose testing), trophic changes, limitation of mobility in metacarpophalangeal, proximal and distal interphalangeal joints
- Eyes – cataract, squint
- Fundi
  — non-proliferative retinopathy: haemorrhages, exudates and microaneurysms
  — proliferative retinopathy: new vessel formation, vitreous haemorrhage, retinal detachment
- Peripheral neuropathy – predominantly distal sensory loss. Check vibration, position and light touch; ankle reflexes may be absent
- Mononeuropathy – may affect cranial nerves
- Blood pressure – hypertension; postural hypotension if autonomic neuropathy
- Skin – necrobiosis lipoidica (lesions usually on shins; shiny, red or yellowish plaques with tendency to atrophy at centre)
- Injection sites – lipoatrophy or lipohypertrophy

Associations
- Autoimmune diseases, e.g. hypothyroidism, Addison's disease
- Coeliac disease (see p. 31)
- Prader–Willi syndrome (see p. 170)
- Cystic fibrosis (see p. 7)
- DIDMOAD
- Diabetes insipidus, diabetes mellitus, optic atrophy and deafness

Key points

- Incidence in UK is 13.5 in 100 000, with 25% < 5 years at time of diagnosis
- Marked geographical variation with rates increasing with distance from the equator
- Genetic predisposition, with HLA-DR3/4 being strongly associated
- Early recognition of classic signs (polyuria, polydipsia, weight loss) results in most children starting treatment before severe ketoacidosis and dehydration develop
- Maintaining good glycaemic control is important in limiting long-term complications
- A multidisciplinary team approach is required in optimising care

Gaucher disease

Physical signs
- Hepatomegaly
- Splenomegaly
- Yellow-brown pigmentation of the skin
- Ataxia and eye movement disorders (in type II)

Associations
- Skeletal complications, e.g. fractures of femoral neck and vertebral bodies
- Hypersplenism

Key points
- Autosomal recessive inheritance
- Lysosomal storage disorder due to a deficiency in β-glucosidase activity
- Type I patients (adult; more prevalent in Ashkenazi Jews) have hepatosplenomegaly without neurological involvement
- Type II patients (infantile) present early, have neurological involvement and usually die in the first 2 years of life
- Type III patients (juvenile) characterised by neurological regression and seizures
- Bone marrow examination usually shows typical Gaucher cells; diagnosis is made on confirming a deficiency of β-glucosidase in white cells or fibroblasts

Glycogen storage disease

TYPE Ia: VON GIERKE DISEASE

Physical signs
- Small stature
- Rounded face ('doll's face' or 'cherub face')
- Protuberant abdomen
- Hepatomegaly but no splenomegaly
- Kidneys may be enlarged
- Hypotonia

Associations
- Easy bruising and nosebleeds
- 10% develop xanthomata
- Liver adenomata and cirrhosis
- Gout

Key points
- Autosomal recessive condition occurring in 1 in 400 000 live births
- Deficient glucose-6-phosphatase impairs glycogenolysis and gluconeogenesis, resulting in troublesome hypoglycaemia
- Management involves frequent glucose feeds
- Normal mental development
- GSD type Ib, due to a defect in glucose-6-phosphatase transport system, has similar clinical features, but in addition recurrent infections due to neutropenia

TYPE IIa: POMPÉ DISEASE

Physical signs
- Hypotonia
- Progressive weakness
- Absent reflexes
- Hepatomegaly
- Cardiomegaly

Associations
● Cardiac arrhythmia

Key points
● Autosomal recessive disease due to absence of lysosomal α-1,4-glucosidase activity
● Most infants die in the first 2 years of life from chest infection and/or cardiac involvement
● Characteristic ECG with short P–R interval and large QRS complexes
● Type IIb presents with a myopathy in childhood and progresses more slowly

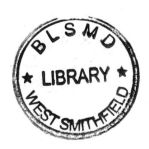

Hyperthyroidism

Physical signs
- Thin but well grown
- Warm skin
- Excessive sweating
- Fine tremor of the outstretched hands
- Tachycardia, wide pulse pressure (check for systolic hypertension)
- Diffuse goitre often with a bruit
- Eyes prominent and staring with lid lag and/or lid retraction
- Exophthalmos may be present
- Proximal muscle weakness
- Shortened relaxation phase of deep tendon reflexes

Associations
- Diabetes mellitus (see p. 132)
- Addison disease
- Down syndrome (see p. 156)

Key points
- Thyrotoxicosis in children is nearly always due to Graves disease and results from the presence of thyroid-stimulating immunoglobulins
- Other rare causes include thyroiditis, iodine toxicity, McCune–Albright syndrome, thyroid neoplams, TSH hypersecretion, thyroid hormone ingestion
- Infiltrative ophthalmopathy is unrelated to circulating thyroid hormone levels; it does occur in children but rarely progresses to muscle paralysis, chemosis and visual loss

Hypothyroidism (with a goitre)

Physical signs
- May have pallor, rounding of the face, periorbital oedema
- Skin is dry and cool
- Hair is sparse and brittle
- Short stature and overweight
- Diffusely enlarged, firm, non-tender goitre
- Pulse rate is slow; may have reduced pulse pressure
- Hypotonia and muscle weakness
- Delayed relaxation phase of the tendon reflexes
- Slowness in speech, thought and movement

Associations
- Diabetes mellitus (see p. 132), Addison disease, hypoparathyroidism
- Turner syndrome (see p. 174), Noonan syndrome (see p. 168), Down syndrome (see p. 156)
- Pendred syndrome (sensorineural deafness, hypothyroidism, goitre – autosomal recessive inheritance)

Key points
- Hashimoto's thyroiditis is the most common cause – diagnosed by biochemical evidence of hypothyroidism and presence of antibodies to thyroid microsomal antigen and thyroglobulin
- Other rare causes include de Quervain's thyroiditis and acute suppurative thyroiditis following haemolytic streptococcal infection
- Treatment is by thyroxine replacement at ~ 100 $\mu g/m^2$ per day adjusted according to clinical response and TSH levels

Mucopolysaccharidosis

HUNTER SYNDROME (MUCOPOLYSACCHARIDOSIS II)

Physical signs
- Affects males
- Proportionate short stature
- Macrocephaly
- Clear cornea
- Coarse facial features – thickening of lips, tongue and nostrils, widely spaced teeth, prominent supraorbital ridges
- Hirsute
- Thick skin; nodular skin lesions may be present on arms or posterior chest wall
- Short neck
- Recurrent rhinorrhoea and noisy breathing
- Umbilical and/or inguinal herniae
- Hepatosplenomegaly
- Joint stiffness
- Intelligence may be normal or mildly impaired in 'mild form'; in 'severe form', mental and neurological deterioration produce profound problems by late childhood

Associations
- Cardiac failure due to mucopolysaccharide deposition
- Myelopathy from meningeal thickening
- Progressive hearing loss and joint contractures

Key points
- X-linked recessive inheritance with an incidence of about 1 in 100 000 live births
- Clinical features and inheritance distinct from Hurler syndrome although both excrete dermatan and heparan in the urine
- Deficient enzyme is iduronate sulphatase
- No curative treatment, and management is largely supportive
- Survival into adulthood, but in the severe form death occurs from cardiac and respiratory problems in the 20s; in the mild form, survival beyond 60 has been recorded

HURLER SYNDROME (MUCOPOLYSACCHARIDOSIS I–H)

Physical signs
- Proportionate short stature
- Macrocephaly
- Corneal clouding
- Coarse facies – depressed nasal bridge, bulbous nose, prominent supraorbital ridges, large tongue and lips, small widely spaced teeth
- Mucoid rhinorrhoea
- Fine body hair
- Hepatosplenomegaly
- Inguinal and umbilical herniae
- Joint contractures, especially the phalanges, elbows, shoulders and hips
- Kyphosis
- Deterioration in mental development

Associations
- Limited vision from corneal clouding and degenerative changes in retina
- Cardiac failure from mucopolysaccharide deposition

Key points
- Autosomal recessive inheritance occurring in 1 in 100 000 live births
- Features due to deposition of acid mucopolysaccharide
- Underlying defect is deficient function of α-L-iduronidase
- Management is largely supportive; bone marrow transplant may be curative
- Cardiac and respiratory decompensation leads to death before 10 years of age in most patients

MORQUIO SYNDROME (MUCOPOLYSACCHARIDOSIS IV)

Physical signs
- Truncal shortening, kyphoscoliosis, exaggerated lumbar lordosis
- Flaring of the lower ribs
- Short curved long bones and short stubby hands
- Joint laxity

- Prominent lower face
- Widely spaced teeth and thin enamel
- Cloudy cornea
- Aortic regurgitation

Associations
- Hypoplasia and subluxation of first and second cervical vertebrae, leading to spinal cord and nerve root compression
- Relatively normal intellectual development

Key points
- Autosomal recessive inheritance
- Deficiency identified in two enzymes: the more severe (type A) results from deficiency in n-acetyl-galactosamine-6-sulphatase; the milder (type B) results from a deficiency in β-galactosidase
- Cardiac and neurological complications limit survival, which is usually into early adulthood
- No curative treatment and management is largely supportive; surgical/orthopaedic intervention (e.g. fusion of cervical spine) may be indicated

SANFILIPPO SYNDROME (MUCOPOLYSACCHARIDOSIS III)

Physical signs
- Macrocephaly
- Mildly coarse facies
- Synophrys
- Mild hirsutism
- Hepatosplenomegaly (develops in school age children)
- Slowing of development – often apparent within 1–2 years with subsequent severe regression

Associations
- Hyperkinesis and aggressive behaviour

Key points
- Autosomal recessive inheritance
- Biochemical defect is in the breakdown of heparan sulphate

- Identification of specific enzyme defects has led to recognition of four groups (A, B, C and D), although clinical features are the same
- Outlook limited by severe impairment resulting from central nervous system involvement

SCHEIE SYNDROME (MUCOPOLYSACCHARIDOSIS I–S)

Physical signs
- Joint limitation, particularly of phalanges, elbows and shoulders
- Genu valgum
- Broad short hands
- Mild facial coarsening
- Corneal clouding
- Inguinal and umbilical herniae
- Check for cardiac murmurs arising from aortic valvular defect

Associations
- Carpal tunnel syndrome
- Blindness from corneal clouding and retinal degeneration

Key points
- Autosomal recessive inheritance
- Results from a deficiency in α-L-iduronidase
- Although there is no curative treatment, it is compatible with normal intelligence and survival into early adulthood

Pseudohypoparathyroidism

Physical signs
- Short stature
- Round face and short neck
- Obese
- Metacarpal and metatarsal shortening, especially the 4th and 5th; results in dimpling on dorsum of hand
- Ectopic calcifications, especially near the joints
- May have delayed tooth eruption and enamel hypoplasia
- Moderate degree of mental retardation
- Chvostek's and Trousseau's signs normal in treated cases

Associations
- The characteristic clinical features referred to as Albright hereditary osteodystrophy
- Hypothyroidism and hypergonadotrophic hypogonadism

Key points
- Autosomal dominant inheritance
- Presentation may be with hypocalcaemic tetany and/or convulsions
- Treatment is with oral calcium supplements and vitamin D analogue
- Pseudopseudohypoparathyroidism – patients have clinical features but not the biochemical abnormalities

Exam syndromes

11

Alagille syndrome

Physical signs
- Proportionate short stature
- Prominent forehead/frontal bossing
- Deep set eyes
- Hypertelorism
- Prominent nasal bridge
- Peripheral pulmonary stenosis
- Signs of hepatic dysfunction, e.g. jaundice and scratch marks from pruritus
- Butterfly vertebrae – check back for any deformities
- Rib anomalies

Associations
- Prolonged neonatal jaundice from intrahepatic bile duct paucity
- Renal anomalies
- Mild mental retardation in ~ 15% of cases

Key points
- Incidence approximately 1 in 100 000 live births
- Inheritance is autosomal dominant with variable expression
- Survival often into adult life
- Treatment includes alpha-tocopheryl acetate, phenobarbitone and cholestyramine
- Neurological sequelae of vitamin E deficiency may occur despite treatment

Angelman (happy puppet) syndrome

Physical signs
- Happy appearance ± inappropriate laughter
- Characteristic arm posture (resembling a puppet)
- Prominent jaw
- Maxillary hypoplasia
- Tongue protrusion
- Widely spaced teeth
- Microbrachycephaly
- Deep set eyes
- Jerky movements
- Hypotonia
- Growth retardation
- Ataxic gait

Associations
- Mental retardation (severe)
- Optic atrophy
- Seizures; characteristic EEG

Key points
- Prevalence of about 1 in 10 000–20 000
- Inheritance is by an absence of maternal contribution to chromosome 15 (15q11–13) due to either a deletion or paternal uniparental disomy

Beckwith–Wiedemann syndrome

Physical signs
- Neonatal macrosomia
- Macroglossia
- Horizontal ear lobe crease
- Small pits behind helix of ear
- Organomegaly – check for enlarged kidneys, liver or spleen
- Omphalocele (look for scar from surgical repair)
- Facial naevus flammeus

Associations
- Neonatal hypoglycaemia due to islet cell hyperplasia
- Accelerated growth and bone maturation
- Diaphragmatic eventration
- Hemihypertrophy

Key points
- Sporadic and autosomal dominant inheritance described
- Unrecognised neonatal hypoglycaemia may result in mental retardation
- Increased incidence of Wilms tumour; hemihypertrophy seen in 40% of those developing Wilms tumour

CHARGE association

Physical signs
- Coloboma
- Heart defect, e.g. patent ductus arteriosus, atrial septal defect, ventricular septal defect
- Atresia choanae
- Retarded growth
- Genital anomalies
- Ear anomalies and deafness

Associations
- Facial nerve palsy
- Mental retardation

Key points
- Diagnosis made if four of the major criteria are present, one of which should be either coloboma or choanal atresia
- Sporadic inheritance
- Choanal atresia – may be unilateral or bilateral with a bony or membranous septum
- Bilateral choanal atresia usually presents in the newborn period due to obstructed breathing

Cornelia de Lange syndrome

Physical signs (Fig. 8)

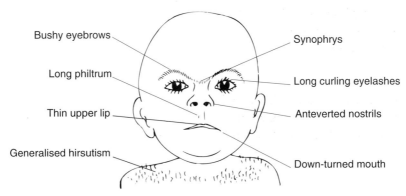

Bushy eyebrows

Synophrys

Long philtrum

Long curling eyelashes

Thin upper lip

Anteverted nostrils

Generalised hirsutism

Down-turned mouth

Fig. 8 Cornelia de Lange's syndrome.

- Short stature
- Microbrachycephaly
- Generalised hirsutism with hair whorls over arms and posterior trunk
- Synophrys with bushy eyebrows
- Small nose with anteverted nostrils
- Long philtrum
- Thin upper lip
- Micrognathia
- Late erupting hypoplastic teeth
- Limb malformation (seen in approximately 25%)
    — micromelia
    — phocomelia and oligodactyly
    — proximal implantation of thumbs
- Simian crease
- Clinodactayly
- Flexion contraction of elbow
- Abnormal genitalia

— hypoplasia
— undescended testes
— hypospadias

Associations
- Mental retardation
- Complex congenital heart disease
- Abnormal hoarse cry
- Seizures (20%)

Key points
- Inheritance is usually sporadic
- Antenatal growth retardation
- Present at birth with multiple anomalies

Craniosynostosis

APERT SYNDROME

Physical signs (Fig. 9)

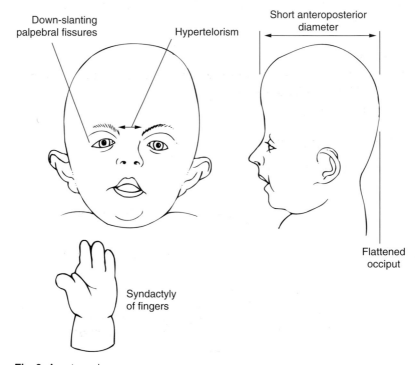

Fig. 9 Apert syndrome.

- Acrocephaly – head is tower-shaped with short anteroposterior diameter, high forehead and flat occiput
- Craniosynostosis – coronal suture most common but also saggital and lambdoid
- It is difficult to differentiate one craniosynostosis syndrome from the others on facial appearances alone. Hence, it is essential to look for associated hand abnormalities
- Flat facies, maxillary hypoplasia, hypertelorism, down-slanting palpebral fissures, shallow orbits

- Syndactyly of fingers and toes, broad distal phalanges of thumbs and hallux
- Cleft palate

Associations
- Mental retardation in about 50% of affected individuals
- Limited joint mobility
- Cardiac defects, raised intracranial pressure, optic atrophy, hearing loss

Key points
- Surgical intervention may be indicated for cosmetic reasons and raised intracranial pressure
- Inheritance is sporadic

CROUZON SYNDROME

Physical signs (Fig. 10)

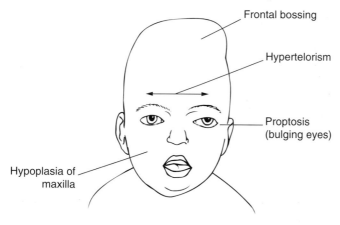

Fig. 10 Crouzon syndrome.

- Craniosynostosis – coronal, metopic and sagittal sutures, frontal bossing, brachycephaly, hypoplasia of maxilla
- Proptosis
- Conductive hearing loss
- Normal intelligence

Associations
- Chiari malformation and hydrocephalus
- Raised intracranial pressure
- Optic atrophy
- Occasional seizures

Key points
- Inheritance is autosomal dominant with variable expression
- Surgical intervention may be indicated for cosmetic reasons and raised intracranial pressure

PFEIFFER SYNDROME

Physical signs
- Brachycephaly
- Craniosynostosis – coronal and sagittal sutures
- High full forehead
- Hypertelorism
- Up-slanting palpebral fissures
- Small nose with low nasal bridge
- High-arched palate
- Broad distal phalanges of thumb and first toe

Associations
- Choanal atresia
- Mental retardation
- Seizures
- Hearing loss

Key points
- Inheritance is autosomal dominant
- Surgical intervention may be indicated for cosmetic reasons and raised intracranial pressure

DiGeorge syndrome

Physical signs
- Hypertelorism
- Short philtrum
- Micrognathia
- Down-slanting palpebral fissures
- Ear anomalies, e.g. notch in pinna, hypoplasia of auricle
- May have cardiac anomalies

Associations
- Cardiac – interrupted aortic arch/conotruncal defect
- Thymic hypoplasia causing T-cell deficiency
- Hypoparathyroidism causing hypocalcaemia ± seizures
- Mild mental deficiency

Key points
- Sporadic inheritance; commonly due to deletion on chromosome 22
- Overlap with velocardiofacial syndrome; termed CATCH 22 syndrome (Cardiac defects, Abnormal facies, Thymic hypoplasia, Cleft palate and Hypocalcaemia) to encompass these similar syndromes
- Abnormal development of 4th branchial arch and 3rd/4th pharyngeal pouches
- Recurrent candidiasis, chest infections and diarrhoea due to the immune deficiency
- Hypocalcaemia is corrected with oral supplements and 1-alpha-hydroxycholecalciferol
- HLA identical bone marrow transplant, if available, is the optimal treatment for the immune deficiency

Down syndrome

Physical signs (Fig. 11)

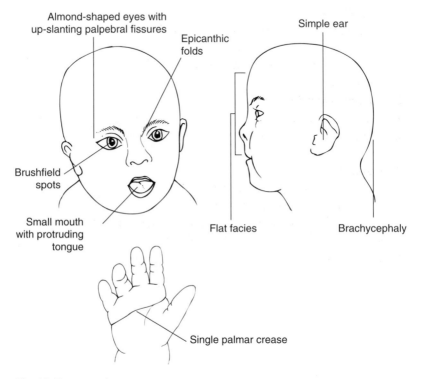

Fig. 11 Down syndrome.

- Up-slanting palpebral fissures
- Epicanthic folds
- Brachycephaly
- Brushfield spots
- Lens opacities
- Small mouth often held open with protruding tongue
- Low nasal bridge
- Single palmar crease
- Short broad hands
- Fifth finger clinodactyly

- 'Sandal' gap between first and second toes
- Hypotonia
- Short stature
- May be centrally cyanosed
- Mental retardation

Associations
- Congenital heart disease – atrioventricular septal defect is characteristic but any lesion may occur
- Increased risk of leukaemia (AML and ALL)
- Dementia
- Duodenal atresia
- Hypothyroidism
- Atlantoaxial instability

Key points
- Trisomy 21 (95%), translocation (4%), mosaic (1%)
- Frequency is 1 in 700 live births
- Increased risk with increasing maternal age – approximately 1 in 900 at 30; 1 in 350 at 35; 1 in 100 at 40 years
- May be antenatally diagnosed on amniocentesis

Ellis–van Creveld syndrome

Physical signs
- Short limbs
- Small chest
- Postaxial polydactyly
- Hypoplastic nails
- Multiple oral frenulae
- Oligodontia
- Cleft lip and palate

Associations
- Congenital heart defects (present in ~40%; atrial septal defect most common)
- Neonatal teeth

Key points
- Autosomal recessive inheritance
- Small chest may cause respiratory embarrassment
- Have wide metaphyses on X-ray

Fragile X syndrome

Physical signs
- Large head with prominent forehead
- Long thin face
- Thickening of nasal bridge
- Prominent jaw
- Pale blue irides
- Large ears; may be posteriorly rotated
- Large testes
- Hypotonia
- Joint laxity
- Characteristic speech 'cluttering'
- Hyperkinetic behaviour

Associations
- Mental retardation

Key points
- Fragile site located on distal long arm of chromosome X
- Clinical manifestations relate to expansion of trinucleotide repeat sequence; an increasing severity of the condition is seen with increased expansion
- The trinucleotide expansion increases with each generation
- Female carriers may also be affected, often mildly

Goldenhar syndrome (oculo-auriculovertebral anomaly)

Physical signs (Fig. 12)

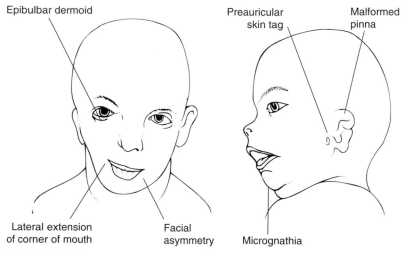

Fig. 12 Goldenhar syndrome.

- Facial asymmetry (hemifacial hyposomia)
- Mandibular hypoplasia
- Hypoplastic zygomatic arch
- Malformed pinna
- Preauricular skin tags or sinuses
- Microphthalmia
- Coloboma of eyelid
- Epibulbar dermoid

Associations
- Deafness which may be conductive or sensorineural
- Cardiac malformations including ventricular septal defect and Fallot tetralogy
- Vertebral anomalies
- Cleft lip and palate

Key points

- Inheritance is sporadic
- Bilateral facial involvement in ~a-third of cases – one side nearly always more severely affected (usually the right)

Holt–Oram syndrome

Physical signs
- Limb reduction defects of variable severity and frequently asymmetrical:
  — phocomelia
  — hypoplastic thumbs
  — triphalangeal thumbs
  — hypoplastic radius
- Also, defects of ulna, humerus, clavicle, scapula and sternum
- Cardiac defects in 85% – atrial or ventricular septal defects are the most common

Associations
- Absent pectoralis major
- Pectus excavatum
- Vertebral anomalies

Key points
- Inheritance is autosomal dominant with variable expression
- At-risk individuals should be investigated with limb X-rays and echocardiogram

Kallman syndrome (hypogonadotrophic hypogonadism)

Physical signs (variable)
- Tall stature, generalised obesity
- Hypogonadism
- Absent secondary sexual characteristics
- Anosmia
- Occasionally cleft lip or palate, choanal atresia, deafness

Associations
- Mild to moderate mental retardation
- Congenital renal anomalies and ichthyosis (in X-linked recessive)
- Increased risk of testicular tumours

Key points
- Isolated gonadotrophin deficiency
- Inheritance variable but usually X-linked recessive
- Presentation in adolescence (delayed puberty)
- Low serum testosterone and prepubertal levels of gonadotrophins, but a positive response to GnRH stimulation
- Treatment is with testosterone replacement and pulsatile GnRH.

Kartagener syndrome (primary ciliary dyskinesia)

Physical signs
- Dextrocardia
- Situs inversus
- Thick nasal secretions
- Chronic sinusitis
- Otitis media; may have grommets
- Bronchiectasis
  — clubbing of fingers (not always)
  — productive cough
  — crepitations over affected lung

Associations
- Cardiac anomalies
- Abnormal neutrophil chemotaxis
- Sterility in males due to sperm immotility
- Conductive hearing loss
- Anosmia

Key points
- Primary defect in microtubules of cilia
- Incidence is 1 in 20 000; autosomal recessive inheritance
- Considerable morbidity due to bronchiectasis
- Treatment symptomatic with physiotherapy and antibiotic therapy
- Prognosis is reasonable in absence of cardiac disease or extensive bronchiectasis

Laurence–Moon–Biedl syndrome

Physical signs
- Short stature
- Obesity
- Polydactyly
- Hypogonadism
- Visual impairment usually in second and third decades

Associations
- Mental retardation
- Retinitis pigmentosa
- Renal defects
- Diabetes mellitus

Key points
- Autosomal recessive inheritance
- Obesity does not present until after infancy but most are obese by 4 years
- Hypogonadism and pubertal failure due to deficiency in gonadotrophins

Marfan syndrome

Physical signs
- Tall and slim
- Arm span > height
- Long thin arms (dolichostenomelia)
- Long and tapering fingers (arachnodactyly)
- Thumb and fifth finger overlap around wrist (wrist sign)
- Thumb extends beyond ulnar border of hand when opposed across palm (Steinberg's sign)
- Joint laxity may result in recurrent dislocation
- Pectus excavatum or pectus carinatum
- Kyphoscoliosis
- High-arched palate
- Eyes
  — ectopia lentis (*upward* subluxation of lens)
  — retinal detachment
  — strabismus

Examine cardiovascular system
- Mitral valve prolapse
  — mid-systolic click + late or pansystolic murmur
- Aortic regurgitation due to root dilatation
  — mild: soft, early diastolic murmur in aortic area
  — severe: cardiac failure, high-volume pulse and displaced apex beat
- Ask to measure BP

Key points

- Prevalence is approximately 1 in 10 000
- Autosomal dominant with variable expression
- Due to mutation of the fibrillin gene on chromosome 15
- Distinguished from homocystinuria by direction of lens subluxation, absence of mental retardation and lack of homocystine in urine
- Regular evaluation with echocardiography for early detection of cardiovascular abnormalities
- Life span may be reduced by cardiovascular complications

Noonan syndrome

Physical signs
- Short stature
- Epicanthic folds
- Downward slanting palpebral fissure
- Ptosis
- Mild hypertelorism
- Deeply grooved philtrum
- Low set posteriorly rotated ears
- Short webbed neck
- Trident hairline (low posteriorly)
- Anterior dental malocclusion
- Pectus excavatum or carinatum
- Shield chest
- Cubitus valgus
- Small penis, cryptorchidism
- Occasional oedema of dorsum of hands and feet

Associations
- Mild mental retardation
- Congenital cardiac defects (80%) – pulmonary stenosis, atrial septal defect, septal hypertrophy
- Vertebral anomalies

Key points
- Usually sporadic inheritance occurring in males and females
- Feeding difficulties commonly reported in neonatal period
- Exclude Turner syndrome mosaic in females, which have a similar phenotype

Pierre Robin sequence

Physical signs (Fig. 13)

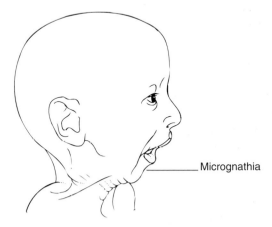

Micrognathia

Fig. 13 Pierre Robin sequence.

- Micrognathia
- U-shaped cleft palate

Associations
- Congenital heart disease
- Feeding problems

Key points
- Sporadic inheritance
- Airway obstruction may result from the tongue falling back into the pharynx (glossoptosis); tracheostomy sometimes required
- The sequence is associated with conditions causing compression or decreased movement in utero
- Good prognosis if feeding/breathing difficulties managed appropriately

---

Prader–Willi syndrome

Physical signs
- Obesity in older child
- Almond-shaped eyes
- Prominent forehead with narrow bifrontal diameter
- Triangular-shaped upper lip
- Hypogonadism/cryptorchidism
- Short stature
- Small hands and feet
- In neonates and infants the major sign is hypotonia

Associations
- Mental retardation, usually mild to moderate
- Hyperphagia
- Diabetes mellitus
- Behavioural difficulties, e.g. temper tantrums, obsessional traits

Key points
- Inheritance due to absence of paternal contribution to chromosome 15 (15q11–13), as a result of either deletion or maternal uniparental disomy
- Reduced fetal movements and breech presentation are common
- Presents in neonatal period with hypotonia, dysmorphism and feeding difficulties
- Failure to thrive in infancy is common before developing marked hyperphagia and obesity

Rubinstein–Taybi syndrome

Physical signs
- Broad or duplicated terminal phalanges of thumb and first toe
- Terminal phalanges of other fingers affected (73%)
- Clinodactyaly of fifth finger
- Mild microcephaly
- Downward slanting palpebral fissure
- Prominent 'beaked' nose
- Broad nasal bridge
- Hypertelorism
- Posteriorly rotated ears
- High-arched palate
- Generalised hirsutism
- Proportionate short stature

Associations
- Mental retardation (most are in mild to moderate range)
- Seizures (28%)
- Glaucoma, coloboma and cataract
- Cardiac anomalies, e.g. ventricular septal defect, patent ductus arteriosus

Key points
- Inheritance is sporadic
- Incidence – rare
- Presentation with feeding problems or developmental delay

Russell–Silver syndrome

Physical signs (Fig. 14)

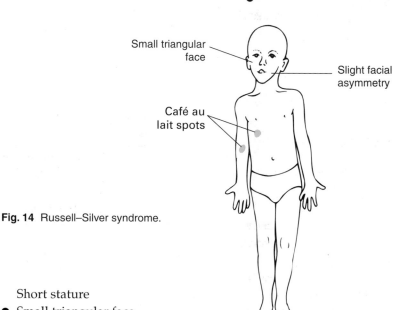

Small triangular face

Slight facial asymmetry

Café au lait spots

Short stature

Fig. 14 Russell–Silver syndrome.

Short stature
- Small triangular face
- Thin lips
- Clinodactyly
- Syndactyly of second and third toes
- Skeletal asymmetry – can involve entire one side of body or be limited, e.g. to a limb
- Café-au-lait spots

Associations
- Small for gestational age
- Precocious puberty

Key points
- Inheritance is usually sporadic; some familial cases have been described
- Consistent abnormalities of growth hormone not demonstrated
- Usually normal intelligence

Treacher Collins syndrome

Physical signs (Fig. 15)

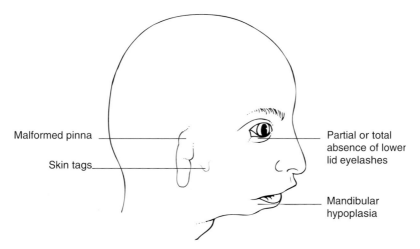

Malformed pinna

Skin tags

Partial or total
absence of lower
lid eyelashes

Mandibular
hypoplasia

Fig. 15 Treacher Collins syndrome.

- Downward slanting palpebral fissures
- Lower lid coloboma
- Partial or total absence of lower eyelashes
- Malar hypoplasia
- Mandibular hypoplasia
- Dysplastic auricles often with skin tags or fistula
- External ear canal defects
- Cleft palate

Associations
- Conductive and sensorineural deafness

Key points
- Inheritance is autosomal dominant with variable expression;
  ~ 50% of cases represent fresh mutations
- Facial abnormalities are usually symmetrical
- Majority of cases have normal intelligence
- Hearing impairment must be detected and treated

Turner syndrome

Physical signs (Fig. 16)

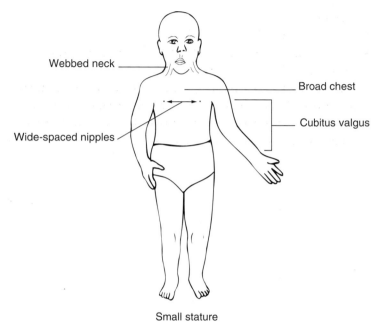

Webbed neck

Broad chest

Cubitus valgus

Wide-spaced nipples

Small stature

Fig. 16 Turner syndrome.

- Small stature
- Low posterior hairline
- Short webbed neck
- Broad chest
- Wide-spaced, often hypoplastic nipples
- Narrow maxilla
- Small mandible
- Cubitus valgus
- Congenital lymphoedema of dorsum of fingers and toes in neonates
- Narrow, convex and deep set nails
- Check femoral pulses and ask for four limb blood pressure

Associations

- Renal anomalies – most commonly horseshoe kidney
- Cardiac defects (20%) – bicuspid aortic valve, coarctation of aorta, valvular aortic stenosis
- Ovarian dysgenesis

Key points

- Incidence is 1 in 3000 live births
- Most common karyotype is 45 XO but mosaics also occur
- Mean IQ ~ 95
- Treatment with oestrogen replacement and growth hormone improves adult height and secondary sex characteristics
- XO/XY mosaicism has increased risk of gonadoblastoma and therefore gonads are surgically removed

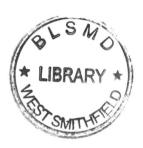

Williams syndrome

Physical signs (Fig. 17)

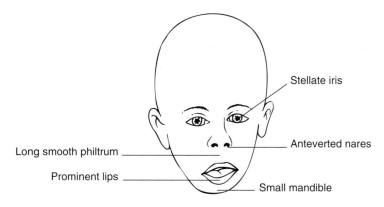

Stellate iris

Anteverted nares

Long smooth philtrum

Prominent lips

Small mandible

Fig. 17 Williams syndrome.

- Small stature
- Elfin features
- Stellate iris pattern
- Periorbital fullness
- Depressed nasal bridge
- Small mandible
- Broad maxilla and prominent cheeks
- Full nasal tip
- Anteverted nares
- Long smooth philtrum
- Partial anodontia and enamel hypoplasia
- Dental malocclusion

Associations
- Mild to moderate mental retardation; mean IQ of 85
- Friendly personality
- Neonatal hypercalcaemia
- Congenital cardiac defects

— supravalvular aortic stenosis is the most common
— others: pulmonary valvular/peripheral stenosis, atrial septal defect and ventricular septal defect
- Hyperacusis
- Renal artery stenosis ± hypertension

Key points
- Inheritance is usually sporadic
- Incidence – 1 in 10 000 to 1 in 50 000
- Low birth weight/growth retardation in the first 4 years
- Some catch-up but ultimately short adult stature

Appendices

Appendix 1: Examination of the cardiovascular system

The following is an approach when asked to the examine the cardio-vascular system. However, listen carefully and follow the specific instructions that may be given to you, e.g. 'examine the praecordium', 'listen to the heart', 'feel the pulse'.

- Introduce yourself to the parent and patient
- Ask permission to examine the system
- Expose and position patient appropriately for his/her age
- Make general inspection
  — age and general health
  — colour – check for central cyanosis
  — comment if there are any obvious dysmorphic features

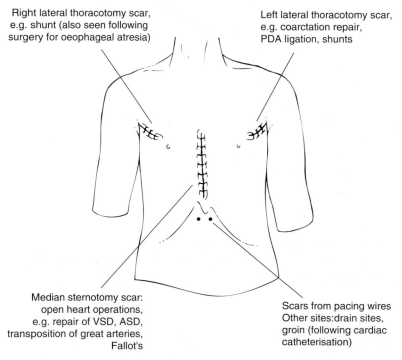

Right lateral thoracotomy scar, e.g. shunt (also seen following surgery for oeophageal atresia)

Left lateral thoracotomy scar, e.g. coarctation repair, PDA ligation, shunts

Median sternotomy scar: open heart operations, e.g. repair of VSD, ASD, transposition of great arteries, Fallot's

Scars from pacing wires Other sites:drain sites, groin (following cardiac catheterisation)

Fig. 18 Scars following cardiac surgery.

- Inspect hands
  — finger clubbing
  — splinter haemorrhages
- Inspect chest
  — operation scars (see Fig. 18)
  — chronic chest deformity
- Check both brachial pulses and femoral pulses – rate, rhythm, character
- Praecordium
  — position and quality of apex beat, thrills including suprasternal notch, heaves
- Auscultate
  — apex (mitral area)
  — 4th intercostal space, left sternal edge (tricuspid area)
  — 2nd intercostal space, left sternal edge (pulmonary area)
  — 2nd intercostal space, right sternal edge (aortic area)
  — *Determine heart sounds*
    — 1st (due to closure of atrioventricular valves)
    — 2nd (due to closure of semilunar valves)
    — 3rd (due to rapid filling of ventricles in diastole)
    — 4th (due to atrial contraction)
    — opening snap, ejection click
  — *Determine murmurs*
    — where loudest
    — timing in cycle (systolic, diastolic, continuous)
    — grade (1 to 6; 4 if palpable thrill)
    — duration (early, late, pan)
    — quality (e.g. harsh, blowing)
    — radiation (neck, axilla, back)
- Lung bases
- Liver
- Brachiofemoral delay in older child
- Say you would check BP – upper limb BP usually 10–20 mmHg less than lower limb BP

Appendix 2: Examination of the respiratory system

Children who are of school age and cooperative can be assessed using a conventional approach as outlined here. The infant and toddler will require a more flexible approach with particular emphasis on inspection at rest.

- Introduce yourself and the examiner to the patient
- Ask permission to examine the system
- Adequately expose and position patient
- Make general inspection
  - age and general health
  - cyanosis
  - other relevant features, e.g. supplemental oxygen, central line, intravenous cannulae
- Hands – check for finger clubbing, examine pulse
- Check tongue for central cyanosis
- Any audible respiratory noises, e.g. stridor, wheeze
- Time respiratory rate (normal range varies with age)
  - newborn: 30–60
  - infancy: 20–40
  - late childhood: 15–25
- Trachea
  - position
  - presence of tracheal tug
- Inspect chest for
  - visible deformities, e.g. pectus excavatum, Harrison's sulcus
  - scars, e.g. thoractomy or sternotomy
  - hyperinflation, intercostal/subcostal recession, chest wall movement
- Apex beat – determine position
- Expansion
- Percussion
  - define areas that are 'dull' or 'stony dull'
  - outline upper border of liver (usually 6th intercostal space anteriorly)

- Auscultation
  - breath sounds: vesicular (normal) or bronchial (consolidation)
  - added sounds
    - wheezes
    - crackles: fine (e.g. fibrosing alveolitis) or coarse (e.g. bronchiectasis, infection)
  - vocal resonance
- Sit forward and examine the back of the chest in a similar sequence
- Additional assessments as relevant may include, for example, peak flow and BP (for pulsus paradoxus)

Appendix 3: Examination of the gastrointestinal system

The following is an approach when asked to the examine the gastrointestinal system. However, listen carefully and follow the specific instructions and if, for example, asked to examine the abdomen then do so.

- Introduce yourself to the parent and patient
- Ask permission to examine the system
- Expose and position patient appropriately for his/her age
- Make general inspection
  - age and general health
  - colour – check for jaundice or pallor
  - comment on nutritional status
- Inspect hands
  - finger clubbing, leuconychia, koilonychia
  - palms for erythema
- Inspect head and neck
  - eyes
  - mouth
- Inspect abdomen – scars, distension, visible veins, stoma
- Palpation
  - assess the four quadrants for tenderness
  - hepatomegaly
  - splenomegaly
  - enlarged kidneys
  - other abdominal masses
  - inguinal lymphadenopathy
- Percussion
  - confirm findings of palpation
  - ascites – test for shifting dullness and fluid thrill if dull in flanks

- Auscultation
- Inspect posterior aspect of abdomen
- Examination of genitalia unlikely to be required in short case section; check whether this is required before proceeding

Appendix 4: Examination of the thyroid gland and thyroid status

You may be required to examine the neck and/or assess clinically a patient's thyroid status.

- Introduce yourself to the parent and patient
- Ask permission to examine
- General inspection
  — age and general health
  — skin colour, hyperpigmentation, vitiligo
  — height and weight
- Examine neck – usually with patient sitting
  — *Inspection*
    — check movement with swallowing
    — size
    — shape
  — *Palpation*
    — tenderness
    — size
    — shape and symmetry
    — mobility
    — lymphadenopathy
  — *Percussion*
    — retrosternal extension
  — *Auscultation*
    — listen for bruit
- Hands
  — thyroid acropachy
  — sweating or dryness
  — tremor of outstretched hand
- Pulse
- Blood pressure
- Eyes:
  — exophthalmos
  — lid lag and/or lid retraction
  — chemosis
  — ophthalmoplegia

- Tendon reflexes
- Proximal muscle strength
- Pretibial myxoedema

Appendix 5: Assessment of short stature

There are many causes of short stature. The most likely explanation may be obvious from general inspection. However, a more structured approach is often required.

- Introduce yourself to the parent and patient
- Ask permission to examine the child
- Make general inspection
  - age
  - colour
  - nutritional status
  - dysmorphic features
  - skeletal abnormalities
  - disproportion
- Inspect hands and upper limbs
  - fingernails
  - palms
  - short 4th metacarpal
  - carrying angle
- Inspect head and neck
  - head
  - hairline
  - ears
  - eyes (including fundoscopy)
  - nose
  - mouth
- Thyroid
- Examination of respiratory, cardiovascular systems and abdomen
- Back
- Lower limbs
- Pubertal staging (if required)

Appendix 6: Examination of the cranial nerves

- Introduce yourself and examiner to the patient
- Ask permission to examine
- Ask patient about change in smell or taste (I)
- Visual acuity (II)
- Visual fields as appropriate for age (II)
- Fundi (II)
- Eye movements (III, IV, VI)
- Nystagmus
- Facial sensation (V, sensory)
- Clench jaws, hold mouth open (V, motor)
- Screw up eyes, look up, blow out cheeks, grin (VII)
- Check hearing (VIII, cochlear) – accurate assessment may not be possible but be prepared to outline approach
- Look at uvula, say 'ah' and watch movement of soft palate (IX, X)
- Observe tongue in mouth, protrude tongue and move side to side (XII)
- Shrug shoulders, turn head and feel sternocleidomastoid (XI)

Appendix 7: Examination of the arms

The approach outlined here may be applied to the older cooperative child but will need adapting depending on age and ability.

- Introduce yourself and examiner to the patient
- Ask permission to examine the system
- Inspection of upper limbs, observing posture (e.g. hemiplegia, brachial plexus injury), deformity, joint abnormalities, skin changes, muscle bulk, fasciculation, involuntary movement
- Tone
- Power (grade out of 5*)
  - shoulder abduction (demonstrate to child elbows flexed and shoulders abducted: C5,6)
  - hold elbows against body (shoulder adduction: C6,7, 8)
  - pull me towards you (elbow flexion: C5,6)
  - push me away (elbow extension: C7,8)
  - wrist extension (demonstrate: C6,7)
  - squeeze my finger (C8, T1)
- Reflexes, using reinforcement if necessary
  - biceps (C5,6)
  - triceps (C7,8)
  - supinator (C5,6)
- Coordination: finger–nose testing, dysdiadochokinesia
- Sensation (assessment of all modalities in short cases not normally required; test light touch in dermatomal distribution and proprioception and proceed to others if indicated)

---

*Grading of power: 0 = no contraction; 1 = flicker of contraction; 2 = movement with gravity removed; 3 = movement against gravity but not resistance; 4 = movement against resistance; 5 = normal power.

Appendix 8: Examination of the legs

The approach outlined here may be applied to the older cooperative child but will need adapting depending on age and ability. Examination of the gait (see p. 192) may be the most appropriate way to start this assessment but is not always possible, e.g. in the severely disabled child.

- Introduce yourself and examiner to the patient
- Ask permission to examine the system
- Inspection of lower limbs oberving posture, deformity, joint abnormalities, skin changes, muscle bulk, fasciculation, involuntary movement
- Tone
- Power (grade out of 5; see p. 190)
  — lift straight leg (hip flexion; L1,2,3)
  — keep leg on bed (hip extension; L5, S1,2)
  — force knee straight (knee extension; L3,4)
  — force knee bent (knee flexion; L5, S1, S2)
  — bend foot up (ankle dorsiflexion; L4,5)
  — bend foot down (ankle plantarflexion; S1)
- Reflexes, using reinforcement if necessary
  — ankle (S1,2)
  — knee (L3,4)
  — Babinski
- Clonus – at knee and ankle ('sustained' is more than three beats)
- Coordination – heel–shin test
- Sensation (assessment of all modalities in short cases not normally required; test light touch in dermatomal distribution and proprioception and proceed to others if indicated)
- Examine back

Appendix 9: Examination of gait

This is a common short case. It may be a lead-in to a more detailed neurological assessment, but also to orthopaedic or rheumatological conditions.

- Introduce yourself to the parent and patient
- Ask permission to examine the gait; this will usually require the child to be undressed to underclothes
- Make general inspection
  — posture
  — deformities and/or contractures
  — muscle bulk
  — neurocutaneous stigmata
- Observe gait and comment if recognisable pattern, e.g.:
  — hemiplegic: circumduction with hip adducted and extended, knee extended, ankle plantar-flexed
  — wide-based: cerebellar pathway
  — waddling: proximal weakness, e.g. Duchenne muscular dystrophy
  — antalgic
- Heel–toe walking
- Other exercises may be helpful in confirming observations, e.g. walking on tip-toes, walking on heels, running, hopping
- If indicated or requested, make formal assessment of lower limbs

Appendix 10: Developmental assessment

6 months
- Pulls to sit (3–6 months)
- Sits with support (4–6 months)
- Sits without support (5–8 months)
- Rolls over (6 months)
- Weight-bearing with legs (3–7 months)
- Parachutes (>4 months)
- Crawls (6–9 months)
- Reaches and grasps rattle (6 months)
- Transfers and mouths (6–8 months)
- Follows fallen toys (6–8 months)
- Plays with feet (6 months)
- Grasps 1 inch cube (watch maturity of grasp)
- Vocalisation (4–6 months)
- Laughs (2–5 months)
- Turns head to sound (4–8 months)

12 months
- Gets to sitting (6–11 months)
- Pulls to standing (6–10 months)
- Creeps (9–11 months)
- Walking
  — holding furniture (7–13 months)
  — alone (10–15 months)
- Points with index finger (11–12 months)
- Casts (9–15 months)
- Pincer grip (9–14 months)
- Holds two bricks and bangs together (7–13 months)
- Knows own name (12–14 months)
- Mama/dada (50% by 15 months)
- Understands several words
- Drinks from cup (10–16 months)
- Plays pat-a-cake (8–13 months)
- Waves bye-bye (8–13 months)

18 months

- Walks backwards (12–22 months)
- Climbs stairs (14–22 months)
- Climbs onto chair (16–18 months)
- Pincer grasp (10–18 months)
- Scribble (12–24 months)
- Tower of 3–4 bricks (18 months)
- Knows three or more words (10–20 months)
- Points to eyes, nose, mouth (14–23 months)
- Obeys simple commands (15–24 months)
- Holds and uses spoon well (17–19 months)
- Takes off shoes (17–19 months)

3–4 years

- Runs fast (3–4 years)
- Climbs stairs in an adult fashion (3 years)
- Pedals tricycle (21–36 months)
- Stands on one foot (22–39 months)
- Hops (3–5 years)
- Walks heel–toe (3–5 years)
- Copies circle (2–3 years)
- Copies cross (3–4.5 years)
- Copies square (4–5.5 years)
- Tower of nine bricks (3 years)
- Copies bridge with three bricks (3 years)
- Sentences of four words (3 years)
- Counts to 10 (3 years)
- Knows full name, sex, age (2.5 years)
- Knows address (4 years)
- Colours (> 3 years)
- Shares toys
- Dresses
  — with supervision (2.5 years)
  — without supervision (> 3.5 years)
- Washes and dries hands (20 months)

Appendix 11: Cover test

General inspection

Squint may be obvious but also comment on epicanthic folds. Get the child's attention and observe the child while one eye is encouraged to focus on a nearby (33 cm) object. Cover the other eye with an occlude or hand. Uncover the occluded eye and observe eye movements whilst covering the other. The squinting eye will move to take fixation when uncovered. Repeat the procedure with a distant (6 m) object.

Range of ocular movements

Test in each eye. In an incomitant motor strabismus, the angle of squint may change and the eyes may be parallel in certain directions of gaze.

Pupillary light reflexes

These should also be tested if 'sensory squint' is suspected. Reflexes are normal if poor vision is due to ambylopia, but they may be abnormal if there is a vision defect due to retinal or optic nerve impairment.

Appendix 12: Distraction hearing test

Sit child on mother's knee facing forwards. The distracter sits in front of the child and the person carrying out the test sounds sits behind the child. The distracter should attract the child's attention with a toy. When the child is alert and attention is focused, the distracter removes the object and stays still. The test sound is then made at about 3 feet away in line and level with the ear. The distracter can then observe the child's response. Repeat the procedure on other side.

Test sounds include low-pitched minimal voice 'ooh' and high-pitched Manchester rattle or minimal voice 'S'. It is important to avoid visual clues and other sensory distractions; hence this test may be difficult to perform in a noisy examination room.

Index

Index